My Dream Mile

My Dream Mile

Charlotte Hagen

The Book Guild Ltd

First published in Great Britain in 2018 by
The Book Guild Ltd
9 Priory Business Park
Wistow Road, Kibworth
Leicestershire, LE8 0RX
Freephone: 0800 999 2982
www.bookguild.co.uk
Email: info@bookguild.co.uk
Twitter: @bookguild

Typeset in Aldine401 BT

Printed and bound in Great Britain by 4edge Limited

ISBN 978 1912575 527

British Library Cataloguing in Publication Data.
A catalogue record for this book is available from the British Library.

Printed on FSC accredited paper

I dedicate this book to the love of my life,
my husband, Stig.

'The man who can drive himself further once the effort gets painful is the man who will win.'

Roger Bannister

★★★

Roger Bannister is an English former middle-distance athlete who in 1954 ran the first four-minute mile; also known as The Dream Mile.

Dear Reader

This book has been written to inspire those of you who have experienced sudden life changes, maybe because of a medical condition that results in a life crisis or any other life-changing event for yourself or your loved ones. It is also written to encourage you to reach out for love, though it seems difficult or even impossible. Mostly it is written to those of you who want to listen. I will admit to you that my story is not unique and neither am I. Today I know that many more of you will have gone through worse situations.

I have no quick or easy solutions about how to deal with a life crisis. I can only hope that my honest story of how I managed my Dream Mile will be of some inspiration to you; that you can use it to grab hold of your life and find the courage to deal with your own situation,whatever may be the cause and fight for your independence. There is only one piece of advice I dare to give to you:

You must remember that inside your changed body, you are still you!

You will discover that although I may not have been

a fast runner I did manage my Dream Mile and it took me all the way to Tuscany in Italy where I live today. I understand now that it has nothing to do with being the one who runs fastest or furthest, but in spite of all the strain and pain, it has everything to do with holding on to your life and being you!

Charlotte Hagen 2018

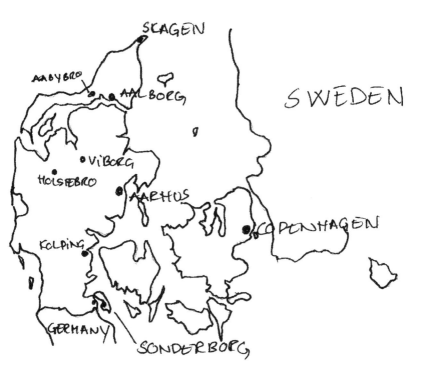

SKAGEN

AABYBRO

AALBORG

SWEDEN

VIBORG

HOLSTEBRO

AARHUS

COPENHAGEN

KOLDING

GERMANY

SONDERBORG

1

It became dark

"I have always dreamt about being in the front of an ambulance driving in an emergency," Jesper whispered to me, followed up by, "so I will be in the front."

I did not remember if I nodded or smiled, I only remember clearly hearing Jesper's words, but not feeling his hand when he touched me gently on my left arm. My body trembled as the paramedics slid the stretcher into tracks in the floor of the ambulance, as they clicked it into place making a stable platform for the patient; in this case, the patient was me. The atmosphere was not very dramatic considering the flashing blue lights and the small crowd that had gathered to watch.

"You don't look very well. We need to take you to the hospital," said the paramedic who was sitting in the back next to me.

I looked over at him and noticed that he had such

trusting eyes. My trembling body relaxed. I felt so calm when I replied to him.

"I have spent most of the afternoon in the hairdressers! You just tell the driver to go up to Hobrovej, turn left and the hospital will be on the right."

These street directions turned out to be the last words I spoke for more than two weeks.

The paramedic smiled at me as the ambulance started its short journey to the hospital. Strange to say I felt so calm and relaxed on the narrow stretcher. It reminded me of when as a little girl I would sit in the back seat of my dad's car as he drove us home from a family visit. The sound of his old car was like a lullaby to my ears and it always rocked me to sleep. Now my brain was begging me to close my eyes and fall asleep.

But the paramedic had decided we were going to talk, so he kept on asking me the same questions over and over again.

"What is your name?"

"How old are you?"

"Where do you live?"

"What is your social security number?"

Surely he could see that I was tired and just wanted to close my eyes and sleep. He was determined that I was going to talk. I felt as if I were a prisoner of war and the enemy was keeping me awake as a form of torture. Eventually, for a few seconds, he stopped talking and I let myself drift into that peaceful world of sleep where I so longed to be.

I woke immediately when I heard the stretcher wheels click, unlatching from their track. The ambulance had parked in front of the emergency entrance of the hospital. As the stretcher and I were being wheeled through its automatic doors I thought, *these doors are to keep the sick in and the healthy out.*

Little did I know how sick I really was.

The bright glare of the lights hanging above my head was too strong for my eyes. I tried to keep them closed so that I could return to the peaceful sleep I had enjoyed for that short period in the back of the ambulance. It was then that I heard the voice of a woman asking Jesper, "What is her name?"

Why was she asking him this? Surely I had given all of this information to the paramedic during our journey here?

Someone then leaned over me and thankfully the glare of the light was blocked from my eyes. Through my blurred vision I could see a man in a white uniform. He looked at me and with a pleasant voice said, "Hello, Charlotte, my name is Frank, I am a doctor. There is nothing to be scared of but I need to drill a small hole into your head."

It was then that the darkness came over me.

2

Memory Lane

It was early afternoon in April of 2014. I had just returned to my home in Lucca loaded down with presents. A few days earlier I had been surrounded by my family and closest friends celebrating my fiftieth birthday in a small cottage just outside of Silkeborg in Denmark.

Dropping my bag just inside the front door I placed the pile of presents on the long dining table in our living room. Everything else had to wait. There was only one thing that occupied my mind at that moment and that was a particular gift from my mum. From my handbag I pulled out a CD. It was a digitalised version of an old VHS video made by my friend Lotte. The CD contained an interview she had done with me more than twenty-two years ago while studying journalism. I was so curious to see what was on that recording that I quickly slipped it into my laptop and sat back to watch.

A picture of me as a young twenty-eight-year-old woman appeared on the small screen. Just looking at it brought memories flooding back. The interview on the disc made me smile, mostly because of what I was wearing and doing. In one scene I was walking on a StairMaster. I was wearing tight white leggings and a neon green top. My flame red hair was long and curly just like Madonna's. It was the late 1980s and it was the height of fashion then. The title of Lotte's film was *The Second Life*, and the theme of the interview was life after a near-death experience. As Lotte was such a good friend to me I had said yes to her.

Recording began in the living room of our house in Viborg. The room had a large picture window overlooking the surrounding forest. I always felt as if we were living in the middle of nature. For the first part of the interview I was sitting on a blue couch with my back to the window. Lotte's fellow student operated the camera. As she got into position and switched on the camera I tried to focus on the small red light above the lens. "How shall I begin?" I asked.

"Just tell me who you are," she replied. So I began.

"My name is Charlotte Hagen and I am a twenty-eight-year-old disabled woman."

I still remember the feeling that hit me when these words came from my mouth. I was surpised by my own reaction. Hearing them filled me with a warmth and tranquillity that I did not expect. Without a doubt it was a true representation of me. Even so, I hated the thought of it. I did not want to be known as 'the disabled woman'. It had been three years since I had had a brain haemorrhage, but even so I was confused by my own words. Today I understand it was because I had not fully accepted the facts about my situation. Filming continued with me exercising in a fitness centre and working in the school at the rehabilitation department of the local hospital in Viborg.

When the CD finished I felt exhausted and a little sad. I wanted to hide it away in my private box, a place where I would keep things that meant a lot to me. This box is made of iron and is always kept in the back of our storeroom. Bringing out the box from its hiding place I placed it on our bed. It took a bit of searching before I found the key to the small lock and it was only when I opened it I realised I had forgotten just how much of my life it contained. Out came a pile of handwritten love letters, old high-school diaries, photographs and a specialist statement from a neuropsychologist.

Unwillingly I was confronted by a long-forgotten, or maybe if truth were told, a more hidden part of my life. As I laid my head back onto the soft pillow I picked up the first photograph. It was me as a young, slim woman. I was on the beach and was topless. According to the writing on the back it was the summer of 1988.

Putting it down I picked up a second photograph taken in the summer of 1989. It was still me but looked like a totally different person. Instead of long, wavy hair, half of my head had been shaved bald. My head was wrapped in bandages and I was sitting in a wheelchair with support to hold my head. I had a wry smile on my face and was drooling a bit from the left side of my mouth.

A sudden feeling of weariness enveloped me and my body became very heavy. Closing my eyes I let myself be dragged into that dark tunnel where time and place did not exist. Now my eyes were too heavy to open and I had to let go of control. I was in the embrace of sleep somewhere between dreams and reality. It was as if I were a third party in their playful dance where dream and reality were trying to take over me. I was disturbed by a sound. Where was I? Asleep or awake?

My conscious mind was trying to give me an answer. I remembered that on a spring day in 1989 I went to visit a friend named Debora. We had planned for me to stay the night in her apartment with her and her beautiful daughter, Louise. I was going out for dinner with a friend in Aalborg and Debora's apartment was closer than travelling back home to my place late in the evening. Even though it was April, the early spring weather was cold and windy so I had to wear a warm jacket over my slim-cut jeans and a favourite white shirt. Trying to keep warm I peddled as fast as I could on my bike from the private school in Åbybro where I was working to my hairdresser nearby and then on to Debora's. I was very happy with my new-look haircut and keen to show it off, so I rode the twenty kilometres to Aalborg very fast.

I arrived at her apartment on the boulevard in Aalborg exhausted. After cups of tea and a girly chat, I made use of her bedroom for a short rest before getting ready to go out. Her room was on the first floor of the house and I could hear the chatter of Louise and Debora from the room underneath. When I woke up there was no sound coming up through the floorboards. I supposed they had decided to take a nap. I felt a sharp pain in either my head or neck and thought that I needed to change my position, or at least move the pillow from underneath. I could not open my eyes. My body felt heavy as if it were cased in concrete and I was sinking down into and through the mattress. I was still so tired I decided to stay on the bed and sleep a little longer.

Suddenly I could hear voices – some clear and others not so. These voices came and then faded away before returning again and again. The only voice that I could clearly distinguish was that of my mum. It sounded as if her voice was floating over me, speaking to me in that familiar soft, gentle tone that I remembered her using when I was a child.

Every time another voice spoke she stopped talking only to start again when the other person was silent. It was nice to listen to her telling me how she gave birth to me in March 1964. She spoke of my early childhood, when I spoke my first words, when I took my first faltering steps and when I started my first day of school. But I had no idea why she was telling me all of this.

The muttering of other voices eventually became clearer to me. It was as if I was in a plane and the altitude had made my ears pop. I swallowed hard and eventually managed to clear them. The voice trying to wake me was not that of Debora but a stranger. "If you are Charlotte then squeeze my hand," the voice of a woman said. I did but she just kept on repeating herself.

3

I know who I am

My name is Charlotte. That I am sure about. I have been Charlotte since I was four years old. It was about the same time I understood that we all have different names.

My mother's name is Dora and my father's name was Børge. I was born and raised in the little town of Løgstør by Limfjorden in the northern part of Denmark. I am also the straggler of two other siblings. My mum gave birth to me in our house on a spring Sunday in 1964. I was born with exactly the same colour hair that she had, although it did not stop her from saying to the doctor as he handed me over to her,

"Red hair! She is ugly." Later in my life she kept telling me that I was beautiful with my red hair.

My big brother's name is Peter and he is ten years older than me. He left home when I was eight years old to join the army. Military life suited his temperament.

He is still responsible and a perfectionist. As the firstborn son he carried the high expectations of our parents. Later I was to learn that my parents had given him a very strict upbringing. After a long and very successful career in the Danish army he resigned his commission and took a job in the energy sector in finance and administration. Divorced from his first wife, he eventually met Marie whom he later married.

Vibeke is my sister, although she has always been known in our family as Vibsen. She was born six years after my brother and four years before me. I think that she felt a little squeezed between the eldest son and the spoilt little sister. Always the princess of the family she knew and still knows exactly how to dress well and is very feminine, unlike me. Vibsen worked in the local jewellery shop. When she married and her husband was offered a job in France they made the move. Since then she has devoted her life to the role of mother and supportive wife.

Then comes me. Whereas both my siblings are tall and slim, I was the chubby little tomboy with the shocking thatch of rust-red hair and freckles. No matter how hard my mum tried I always dressed in jeans topped by a baggy sweater and sneakers. You might think that my look would have been enough to invite some of the local children to bully me but they never did. Probably because they had heard the stories that people with red hair had fiery tempers to go with it! I have never been afraid to speak my mind whether to friends, family or strangers, young or old.

As the last child born of the family I was lucky to have parents who had lived out their dreams with the firstborn, a son, and then the princess. I think that by the time I was born my parents were much more relaxed with my upbringing, more so than with my brother and sister. My parents had gained more control over their own lives and were settled at home and at work. They had more time and energy to enjoy life with their little family.

Unfortunately this did not prevent my mother from developing an exaggerated need to protect and look after me. Several times in the first five years of my life I spent time in hospital due to blood and skin problems. I can only recall one particular moment from all the times in hospital. It was a sunny morning and my mother took me to the hospital and told me to play with the other children and toys in the paediatric department. Suddenly I realised that she had left. I remember that I felt alone and that she had abandoned me. It turned out she had left only to talk to the doctor. Later she returned with my father to visit me. It never took away the hated feeling of being left alone. As predicted by the doctors I grew out of the problems and for a short while Mum was a little less protective.

I was raised in a working-class home. My father worked as a driver at the local sawmill and Mum was a hardworking waitress in a local restaurant. They were both well known in my home town – my mum for being the red-haired waitress always in high heels. The restaurant was the place where everyone in town went to celebrate family occasions like weddings, baptisms and birthdays.

My father was a tall, big, dark man with whom you could always stop and have a chat; maybe share a cold beer with whilst he was emptying his eel traps or working on his vegetable garden. I am certain that he fulfilled many of the preconceived ideas of the people of Jutland. He would rather not leave his hometown, but if for some reason he had to, he first would hide his money in his garden or even under the mattress of his bed. He was a man who lived for his spare time, a real country man who loved the outdoor life of fishing, hunting or just pottering about in his garden.

Some people would say that was the only thing to do in our little town in the northern part of Jutland far from the capital of København. It was not an inspiring place for me, or any other adventurous teenager. We all dreamed of travelling, meeting new people and having exciting adventures.

My chance to escape came when I was admitted to college in the nearby town of Fjerritslev. My parents were so very proud because I would be the first in our family to attend college. I could feel the great weight of expectation coming from my parents especially when my mother told people that maybe I would go on to study law at university. There was no doubt that they only wanted what was best for me, although their expectations just put more pressure on my shoulders. All I really wanted was the freedom to join in the social life of college.

Being at college would not be easy since I lived at home so I asked my parents if I could move away and live closer to the college. That was something they did not approve of and there were many hours of discussions and plenty of stubborn sulking from me before we came to a compromise. I would be allowed to leave home on condition that I moved into my brother's house in Holstebro and finished college there. It turned out to be a good compromise as Peter and his first wife gave me enough freedom and did not act as if they were a second set of parents to me. The price I had to pay for living as a semi- independent young woman was that I had to follow a few reasonable rules in their home and attend college every day.

During that period of my life I dressed a bit like a punk. I was always in old camouflage trousers bought from a military-style store, baggy home-knit sweaters and red boots. I soon gravitated to a group of similarly clothed girls. We basically became a girls' group, meeting in the college canteen, and we discussed philosophy and revolution over cups of herbal tea. We differed from the mainstream student body by our clothing as most of the boys had well groomed, shortish hair and the girls big Madonna curls. We were an odd sight when you saw us all together during our lunch breaks in the canteen.

It was there that I saw Kristian for the first time. He had a sort of bad-boy look. He often ran his fingers through his light blonde hair to brush the fringe from his eyes. Looking around I could see that plenty of other girls had noticed him as well.

I had only been at the college for a week when I saw him. He was sitting having lunch with a boy from my class, named Esben. They were at one end of a long refectory table which our class used every day. I was seated next to one of the girls I had met on my first day and I tried to focus on what she was telling me but my gaze kept wandering over towards Kristian. Firstly I noticed his long blonde hair because he kept running his fingers through it. From where I was sitting it looked like he had quite an athletic body with his long legs stretched out in front of him as he slouched in his chair. When he looked up over at the clock on the wall it was his intense grey-blue eyes that grabbed my attention. Day-old stubble covered his lower face giving him a very photogenic look, baggy trousers and sweatshirt finished it off. His appearance was one of casual tough but with a hint of haunted vulnerability in his eyes.

Suddenly I was brought back to reality when my friend said to me, "Forget him, he is dating one of the senior girls here." I felt a blush rise to my face embarrassed to be discovered staring over at him.

"He is so beautiful to look at but there is a sad look in his eyes," I replied without looking at her.

"That's true! They say that he had a tough time growing up."

I don't think that he noticed me until we met two years later after finishing college.

4

Almost awake

A hoarse, snorting noise woke me. It was terrifying to hear and sounded like a person struggling to breathe, fighting for breath and life. One part of me thought it was the scariest sound possible, the other part that it was a vital sound as it reassured me that I was alive. I could also hear other sounds; some were like a school orchestra tuning before a concert, some were going 'Bip bip' and others 'Bling bling', not scary but stressful. These background noises were mixed with voices. I was listening intently trying to separate the noises and the voices. Eventually I recognised the soft tones of my mother, the deeper ones of my father and brother. I also thought that I could recognise the voice of Kristian, my boyfriend. That confused me. He was supposed to be in København. Sometimes voices of strangers called out measurements or figures, interrupting these familiar voices. There was no longer any doubt. I was not sleeping. This unknown world that I was now inhabiting was the real world for me. I was not at Debora's home safe in bed. I knew because a voice had just told me that I was a patient in the hospital of Aalborg.

The number of different voices that I could hear seemed to have increased. I could hear a lot of muttering. One female voice in particular said, "Charlotte, it is time for you to try to breathe yourself. Do not be scared when you feel us pull a respiration tube through your throat."

I had no idea what she was talking about. I did feel something coming up through my throat and the stinging sensation as it left my body. Someone now touched the side of my face and said. "Well done, Charlotte!"

The noise level in the room dropped and all of the voices I thought I knew disappeared. I guessed it to be midnight. I didn't know as my eyes still refused to open. I had to remain in the darkness. Then I felt panic. Had I suddenly gone blind?

I sensed that some people were still in the room. I transferred all of my energy into trying to hear what they were saying. I registered that there were two female voices. One did move around as the voice came to me from different directions. She had a light but clear way of speaking and to my ears she sounded a bit bossy. She called out various numbers. The second female voice repeated them as if she was trying to memorise them. After a short break the bossy voice said to the second nurse, "In the morning we will remove the feeding tube from Charlotte's stomach and try to give her some proper food. One of the nurses from the day team related that Charlotte loves yogurt and prefers the orange one. If we give her that we can crush her tablets and mix them in with it. Hopefully she will think its muesli and just swallow them."

I could feel myself getting really angry with these two women; I tried to raise my hands to remind them that I was in the room. I wanted to tell them I could hear what they were saying. I tried to send a massive flow of signals from my brain to my arms, but nothing happened. My arms refused to move. I was obviously trapped inside my body. I was now not only angry but extremely frustrated. What was happening to me? To calm myself down, I told myself that as long as I could hear and understand what they said about me, I would be okay. Without knowing what okay would mean, I drifted off to sleep.

Again voices seeped into my brain and I slowly woke up.

"Charlotte, we are going to remove the feeding tube from your stomach. Then we will try to give you some ordinary food to eat. We'll start with something soft and easy to swallow."

I did not realise that I had a feeding tube inserted in me but then again I did not feel hungry.

The nurse gently eased the tube through my nose and I felt the sharp sting as the end worked its way through my throat. Everything seemed to be going so well and quickly and the second nurse from earlier didn't bother to tell me what was going to happen, that she was going to spoon-feed me. As soon as a spoon was pushed between my lips I started to cough and splutter spraying orange yogurt and crushed pills over me, the bed and the surprised nurse. I could hear her walking away muttering to herself. A while later she returned with another yogurt, a new spoon and no doubt more crushed pills. I could not suppress the giggle inside me. This time I hoped she would think twice before trying to put food into my mouth without warning me first. She did and said, "Charlotte, I have a new pot of yogurt and spoon and would like to give some to you now."

Like the good girl that I was I opened my mouth to accept the offering. It was wonderful to feel the cold creamy yogurt in my mouth as it eased slowly down my parched throat. I was certain that this was a whole-milk yoghurt and not my usual low-fat one. It was delightful even if it had a slightly metallic taste of crushed pills.

I could hear the sound of my parents as they entered my room. Mum praised me loudly, "Oh, Charlotte, how wonderful. You are able to breathe by yourself." She did this in the same way that she always used to – highlighting her children's skills in a loud and proud voice. "It is so wonderful to see your progress. You are not only without the machine but you are also trying to eat!"

I thought to myself the pleasure was all hers! Here I was lying in bed covered in orange yogurt, unable to move or even open my eyes and with a sore throat from the tube – some progress.

I had no doubts about anything when I felt the soft touch of my mum or my dad's larger callused hand. I felt them gently touch my cheek, their sense of love and concern in the caress. Suddenly the quiet, peaceful calm of the room was shattered. The door opened and I felt the energetic whirlwind burst in. I could hear the quick clicking steps of stiletto heels approach my bedside. A not so warm hand swept across my cheek. The thought in my head was, *Shit! Things must be serious if Vibsen has come all the way from France to see me.* With her hand now rested on my cheek her internal heating was turned on and her hand started to get warm. Gently I felt her leaning in close to my ear as she whispered, "Hey, sis, please get better soon." The intensity of her emotion was soon broken when she pulled her hand away and started telling my parents how she lost her suitcase in the airport in Paris. Yes, that was the princess for you, Vibsen was in the house. Still trapped inside my body with no language I could not take part in any of the conversations around me. So, for a while, I just shut the world out and took a rest. Peace was restored as my family said goodbye and promised to return again soon.

Shortly after everyone had left, I heard the door open again. Much to my relief it was not doctors or nurses. The voice of my friend Tine said, "Hi, Charlotte, I am here with Anders to visit you."

I did not understand why but she quickly undressed her eight-month-old son and after pulling back my bedclothes laid his naked body onto my stomach before gently covering us both again. But I understood and felt how his little warm body filled me with new life and energy. I could feel a tear roll down the side of my cheek because of this beautiful and generous gift.

I had only known Tine for a few years but it felt so much longer. Never before in my life had I known such a woman, so right for being a mother. She was open-minded, caring and warm with a natural empathy for people. She instinctively knew the right thing to do at the right time. Just as she did by giving me her son, his warm little body filling me with a strength I had never known before. After a while Tine leaned over to take Anders back and said to me, "Take care; no, do not bother. People around you will take care of you. So you just try to relax."

5

Living a double life

My friend Tine was a typical healthy young Danish woman, a very sporty person. She played a lot of handball and so she had an athletic figure and kept her hair cut short. We had first met at teacher training college a few years earlier. It was a chance meeting, as I had never really planned to become a teacher in the first place. My original plan was that after college I would travel to Switzerland to become an au pair. But as the job I had lined up was cancelled and there was nothing else available for me to do, I was forced to move back into my parents' house. There I passed the time working as a cleaner in the local library and in the evenings as a waitress in the restaurant where my mother worked.

On the days I was not cleaning the library I would often visit my grandparents' home with my mother for tea and a chat. On this occasion I took with me a book entitled *What can I be?*. Sitting down close to my grandmother she took the book from me as I poured out the tea. She flicked through the pages until she came to the chapter 'Teaching as a profession'. She pointed to the page, looked up at me and said, "This is your new profession."

I gave her a short laugh and replied, "I do not want to teach other people's badly behaved children!"

My grandmother, a woman who I always thought to be wise and understanding, totally ignored my reply. She just looked back at me. 'It was as if she had lost all sense of hearing.

Again she pointed to the page and said one word, "Teacher!"

I was not going to give in easily and so I tried another argument: "The teacher training college term already started in August. The calendar on your wall says we are now in September."

My grandmother raised herself from her chair and in silence she left the table. I took a deep breath and let out a sigh of relief and carried on flicking through the pages. Yes, I thought I had won! But no. Grandmother was not to be defeated so easily. She returned to the table, put down the telephone and passed the receiver over to my mother with a look that confirmed that mother and daughter had decided my future. Mum dialled the number that was being pointed out to her from the telephone directory. The number turned out to be the direct link to the headmaster of the training establishment in the nearby town of Ranum. He explained that as there was a possibility that the college would be closed by the minister for education, as a cost-cutting exercise, the college had fewer trainees this year. So it would not be a problem for them to accept me as a late entrant. In the end, Grandmother had her own way.

I started teacher training and met Tine. A year later the college closed and we all transferred to other colleges. Tine and I decided that we would go to Aalborg. Tine took the lease on a small one-bedroom apartment just across the bridge that linked Aalborg to Nørresundby, the small town where she was raised. Even though it was only a small apartment Tine asked if I would like to share it with her. I moved in with only my personal belongings, clothing and books. I never really got around to unpacking completely and so my belongings sat around in bags and boxes becoming part of the decoration in the living room. At night I either slept on the living-room sofa or shared the bed with Tine. For the first time in my life I felt freedom. I loved my life in the bigger town with all of its opportunities.

At the weekends we would often hang around in the local bars and pubs on the infamous 'Jomfru Ane Street'. It was on one of these weekends that I saw Esben a former classmate, talking to another young man standing with his back to me. As the young man moved round slightly I recognised his profile. It was Kristian. Leaving my group of friends I walked over to say hi.

At first they did not recognise me. I had changed quite a bit since we last were together. My teenage puppy fat had disappeared as a result of changing my diet. Now

I was eating healthy food instead of too many chocolates and sweets. I was also partaking in an exercise regime prepared for me by Tine. I was now a more feminine and curvaceous young woman. Kristian saw me first. He looked at me but addressed Esben

"My God, surely this cannot be the cheeky little Charlotte from college?"

I did not bother to answer him but rather gave him a slow, provocative look through half-closed eyes. Starting at his feet I worked upwards assessing him and his qualities as a man. Sure enough he had not changed much since I last saw him on graduation day. He was still the same tall, athletic young man with the clear grey-blue eyes, the long hair combed back from his forehead. Now it actually showed a slight receding hairline. Nonetheless, he was still very good-looking. Maybe he was available, as there was no sign of a girl hovering around him. My changed look and attitude must have had a profound effect on him. He looked me over giving me a broad smile as he did so.

"Hi, what are you doing in Aalborg?" he asked, this time addressing me.

"I live in Nørresundby and I am in the second year at teacher training college," I replied.

Kristian pointed at an empty table for two and we went over and sat down. When we left, Esben just said, "See you!" We sat and Kristian started to talk.

"Esben and I are sharing a big apartment on the boulevard. I am studying to be a civil engineer."

His words were not really a great surprise to me as I

had already heard that he was very focused on what he wanted as a career.

We began dating and soon after became lovers. We found that we shared many common interests such as living a healthy lifestyle. Just as importantly, we both had targeted ambitions for our futures.

It was during my final year at the training college that I managed to get a permanent placement at a new private school which had recently opened in Åbybro, about twenty kilometres from Aalborg. The school and its dedicated parents offered me the opportunity to use an alternative approach to teaching. I could use the physical world to give the children a palpable understanding of letters and words. For me it was the responsibility I had for the development of my pupils that I loved. As my ambitions grew I worked all the harder to encourage them and open them to the world.

My work gave Kristian and me an economic opportunity to move away from the city. We rented a small house in the countryside. I now had a boyfriend, a house and a job that I really enjoyed. I felt that my life was close to perfect with the possibility of having a child of our own. Kristian showed no such desire and so I put that dream on hold. Also, he was not even looking for employment of his own. He decided that after he had finished his education in Aalborg he would accept a position at the Danish Technical University in København.

Kristian moved out of our home and into the dorm there. I didn't like to live in our house alone, so I gave up the lease and rented a small apartment close to the school where I was working. For the first few months we flew between the two provinces to spend as much time as possible together. But the plane fares were becoming too expensive and I had to take on a second job just to be able to afford our long-distance relationship. I found one at a bar in Aalborg where at least I could put my waitressing experience to good use. Kristian was so busy with his PhD and I was working so much that we hardly had any time for ourselves.

Most Fridays I would go straight from school into Aalborg where I could stay with various friends before going to work in the bar. Saturday, I would return to their apartments to shower and change clothes before going back for another shift at the bar. Sunday morning, I always took an early bus home. Often I was so exhausted I fell asleep on the bed only to wake up late Sunday evening or early Monday morning. I prepared myself mentally and physically for another week at school, and work life became very difficult for me. I was living a double life. I was tired but I managed because I was young and believed I would live for ever.

On weekdays I was the dedicated teacher with the ambitious boyfriend studying in København. But at the weekend I had a more shadowy and exciting life in the bars and social environment of Aalborg. Eventually I realised that at the weekends my days were shorter and the nights longer.

My dream of a comfortable life with a husband and children began to crumble. Even though Kristian spent more of his time in København doing whatever it was that he did, our relationship changed but we did not break up. He was so occupied with thoughts of his career. He started to talk of moving on to the USA to further his studies. Maybe in hindsight I should have known that his plan was eventually leading to him leaving me. Instead, I told myself that if I was patient and just waited long enough for him to fulfil his professional dream he would come back and we could carry on from where we left off.

6

I am here too

It might be night. The only voices that I could hear were those of the two female nurses from the previous night. I now knew their routine. The first nurse called out a number and the second nurse repeated it. On this night the first nurse stopped what she was doing and said to her colleague, "Last night on our way home from work I kissed him in the lift."

The other nurse replied, "Oh my God, what will you do now?" Then a short pause.

"I don't know. As long as my boyfriend at home never finds out I'll enjoy it." Hearing her words was like having a bucketful of iced water thrown in my face. I started to remember that I had been out having dinner with a new friend. His name was Jesper. I was lying here desperately trying to remember what else had happened to me. I was so very confused.

It was at the birthday party of the sister of my friend Debora two weeks before that I had seen Jesper for the first time. The party was in Debora's small basement flat and when I arrived the party was in full swing. Many young people were talking and wandering around. Candles were on all of the flat surfaces and gave a soft glow to the rooms. In the kitchen a buffet table was covered in various types of Danish foods and a table was overloaded with bottles of beer and wine. I helped myself to some food and picked up a beer before making my way back to the front room to find an empty space to sit. In the end I found a spot on the floor and sat down in front of the sofa. Everyone was talking and I had to raise my voice to introduce myself.

"Hi, I am Charlotte, a friend of Debora's from the teacher training college." One of the boys on the sofa looked over and down at me seated on the floor and said, "I didn't think anyone wanted to be a teacher any more." Normally I would not have given him a second look if we were passing on the street. But his voice just sounded so soft and gentle when he spoke to me. I was surprised that it carried over the conversations of the other party guests. He was sitting on the far end of the sofa and I noticed immediately that he had glorious round, rosy cheeks. He had short, neatly cut brown hair and was fashionably dressed in blue denim jeans and a pale blue polo shirt complete with a little crocodile motif embroidered on the left of his chest. I looked up to his face and directly into his cornflower-blue eyes trying to understand what he meant. He gave me a smile and introduced himself: "Hi, I'm Jesper. Both my parents are teachers and at home they often speak of how few people want to be teachers these days." For some unknown reason I felt an immediate rapport with him. Eventually I discovered that he was equally as argumentative as I was and that we shared the same rather strange sense of humour. Even though I was not totally receptive to his boyish charms, later on in the evening he started to flirt with me, I just went along with it enjoying his attention. By the end of the evening we shook hands to say goodnight. We did agree to meet the following evening at the cinema to watch the film of the moment – *Pretty Woman*.

The visit to the cinema did not cause any further intimate contact. By the time we went our own separate ways we had exchanged contact details, in case either of us needed a companion for a visit to the cinema. It was four days later that Jesper phoned me. At first we talked about various things in general. He suddenly and awkwardly changed the subject.

"Do you want to have dinner with me next week? We can meet at the small Greek restaurant just round the corner from Debora's flat."

I didn't even think before I answered, "I would love to. The twelfth is best for me." My brain was not working but I found myself smiling.

"Perfect. See you on the twelfth at seven," he said and hung up.

The next day I found myself making sure that my skinny black jeans were washed and that my favourite white shirt was ironed. I telephoned Debora to ask if I could use her flat to change before going out, and then stay the night afterwards. The next morning I even made an appointment at the hairdresser.

7

Bang and Babu

At precisely seven o' clock on 12 April 1989 I walked into the Greek restaurant and sat down on the bench opposite Jesper.

When we each had a glass of beer in front of us, Jesper raised his to toast me.

"To health," he said and smiled in that maybe-romantic kind of way.

"Last year, while having dinner in this exact restaurant, I got sick," I blurted out.

"What happened?"

I smiled back before telling him the story. "I had dinner here with some friends. During the main course, I felt a sharp pain in the right side of my stomach. One of our friends rushed me to the emergency department of the local hospital. After a quick examination a doctor informed me that I had an inflamed appendix. I needed to have immediate surgery." I continued coyly, "I hope that the waiter doesn't recognise me," and took a quick look around.

Laughing loudly the only response from Jesper was, "It must have been dramatic."

"It sounds worse than it was, but I pulled through."

On some of the walls in the restaurant there were huge blown-up photographs of long golden sandy beaches, blue-green olive groves and vineyards heavy with plum-coloured grapes. There were photographs with pretty villages complete with little white churches and sky-blue tiled domes representing the heavens. The furniture in the restaurant was painted bright blue in an attempt to convince its patrons they were sitting in a little tavern close to the Aegean Sea. All of these pictures were so overblown you could almost count the grains of sand and the olives on the trees. Anyone who had ever visited Greece would notice a world of difference between this little tavern with its small farmhouse windows in cold Aalborg, Denmark, and the real thing in warm Greece. Greek music was playing a little too loudly for background noise and the suntanned waiter was a little too old to be walking around with his white shirt unbuttoned showing an excessive amount of chest hair.

It was then I heard a loud bang. It sounded as if a balloon had exploded just behind my head. Turning quickly I looked over my right shoulder to see what was happening. All I could see was a white wall. I turned back to face Jesper and gave him a confused look. Once again he laughed while saying, "It's only a wall." Of course, he was right. Behind me there was nothing but a plain white wall.

Without saying anything I got up and went to the bathroom. While washing my hands I looked up into the mirror and was very satisfied with myself and my new haircut. I felt good.

Back at the table I called over to the waiter. "We are ready to order." My voice shocked me. It sounded as if an old-fashioned tape recorder was playing at a low speed and the tape was twisted and dragging through the machine. I knew that there was something seriously wrong happening to me but I had no idea what it was and strangely enough I did not feel frightened. From somewhere in the depth of my memory, I vaguely remembered my grandfather telling me that his voice had sounded strange just before he had had a stroke. The world seemed to stand still for me. I slowly turned to face Jesper and asked, "Do I look or sound weird to you?"

He turned his face to see me. "You look fine!" Then he disappeared from my sight.

"Wait there," I heard him say. I sat alone, stunned. It couldn't have been more than a few seconds before he was back in his chair sitting opposite me. I saw his face clearly now and as I smiled at him he grabbed my right arm. Thinking that he wanted to hold my hand I let him take it but he just turned it around and looking at the watch on his own left wrist put his fingers on my pulse.

This is really odd, I thought to myself. *Why is he doing this? He isn't a doctor.*

Looking over Jesper's shoulder, I saw a man in uniform coming through the doors and over to our table. When he started to speak to Jesper I realised that he was a paramedic. He and his colleague behind him were carrying a stretcher. I made an attempt to stand up from my chair, but I was unable to move.

As I lay in a hospital bed, trying to wake up from my coma, what happened next that evening in the Greek restaurant was all coming back to me in a small series of flashbacks. It had been Jesper in the front seat of the ambulance. Where was he now? How was I going to explain all of this to my boyfriend, Kristian. I remembered that Jesper and I had done nothing wrong. We were new friends. We had met to have dinner in a restaurant, but I had made an effort to look good for him, so it must have seemed that we were on a date. Maybe we had flirted a little.

Gently, the paramedics lifted me onto the stretcher and carried me out to the waiting ambulance. Jesper followed behind, carrying my coat and handbag. A few people coming out of the restaurant, or people in the street, I imagin, formed a crowd around the doors of the ambulance as they clicked shut behind me. In the background I heard the sound of the siren of the ambulance saying "Babu, babu."

8

Year one

They came again, the dismembered voices and endless touching by people I did not know. Then I heard the familiar voices and the touch of my parents and sister. All I could hear them say was, "Please wake up, Charlotte!"

Why did they say this? I was awake.

I could feel the frustration boiling up in me. It only got worse when the unknown voices started to repeat their mantra. "Wake up, Charlotte." It made no sense to me. Why did they keep talking and touching me if they didn't think I was awake? I tried to scream at them to make them understand but nothing came out of my mouth.

Another person took hold of my hand. By the size of the hand it had to be a man. I felt the warm breath from his lips as he spoke gently into my ear. He had a calm, pleasant voice, which I recognised and it was the sound of his voice that convinced me that I was not dead. "Hello, Charlotte, do you remember me? My name is Frank and I am your doctor. Can you open your eyes and wake up for me?"

Reader, can I ask you a question? Have you ever tried to undo the clasp of a bracelet you are wearing on the hand you usually write with by using the fingers of your less dominant hand? If yes, then you know it is only after a struggle and a lot of twisting and turning that it suddenly comes free. When the doctor's gentle voice told me to wake up, it was just like the clasp on my bracelet was coming free. Much to my surprise, I could feel my eyes responding to the message that Frank had sent to my brain.

Slowly I became aware of the bright light over my head. I wanted to close my eyes again but managed to force myself to keep them open.

I gazed around the room. The first person I saw was Frank, my tall doctor, in his crisp white coat standing next to my bed. As my eyes began to focus I could see the worried look on my parents' faces. Then I saw my sister, Vibsen and my boyfriend, Kristian. Lastly, I focused on two nurses in the white uniforms.

"Welcome back, Charlotte. You are in hospital and were admitted on 12 April when you were brought into the emergency room. We discovered heavy bleeding on the right side of your brain. You suffered a brain haemorrhage. To ease the pressure we had to perform an emergency operation to save your life," Frank told me in his laconic voice. I looked up at him and I tried to smile to show that I remembered him. Slowly, he continued to explain. "After the operation you were transferred to the intensive care ward where the doctors and nurses have had you under close observation. I have to tell you that you have been in a coma for the last nine days. Today you are being transferred to the neurosurgery department. But before you leave I would just like to check your eyes."

With his thumb and forefinger he opened my eyes and shined the light from his small pencil torch into them. "Your pupils are back to the right size which means the pressure on your brain is almost back to normal again."

I thought to myself, *I am not sure if this is good news or bad news*. I wasn't really sure of anything.

The two nurses unhooked me from the array of machines that had been connected to my body and prepared to transfer me to my new home: Neurosurgery Room Number Seven. Soon our little procession was winding its way through the corridors of the hospital. We were followed closely by my mum, dad, Vibsen and Kristian at the end. The nurses passed both my notes and me over to the new specialist nurses who connected me to a new monitor before they left me with my family.

Once alone, my mother started to explain how worried they had all been about me. Of that I had no doubt because I could see the drawn looks etched on their faces. I could only presume that it was my mother's religious upbringing that had helped her to get through the last nine days. She looked at me with a big smile but also with tears in her eyes.

"Charlotte, get some rest now. We will be back soon."

Outside I could hear my mother asking the nurse what probably worried her most: "Will Charlotte suffer any permanent brain damage?"

The soft voice of the nurse replied, "At the moment they can say nothing for certain. Only time will tell." Brain damage? BRAIN DAMAGE? How was that possible? I could hear and understand everything they said to me. In my head I created a checklist for year one in my new life and could tick off vision, hearing and understanding as working. I would convince them that I was not brain-damaged. I just had to find a way to tell them.

As promised my family did return to sit with me. This time it was my dad who spoke first. "How are you, Charlotte?" Even though I formulated the words in my head and my lips were ready to say them, I had no voice. I could not speak. As hard as I tried the words would not come out of my mouth. Frustration and rage filled me. I was trapped inside my body with no way of communicating to the outside world. I wondered how my family saw me. Did they see me Charlotte or just a lifeless body?

An anger rushed through my body like a river of molten lava spewing from a volcano. I got so frightened particularly when my right arm suddenly moved in a fast and furious ninety-degree swinging action away from my body. It smashed into a bedside table sending a vase with fresh flowers crashing to the floor, along with glasses of juice, a body lotion and my toothbrush which broke. I felt so angry because I couldn't communicate.

Immediately I saw the fear in my parents' faces and I knew that their worst nightmare could be confirmed by this uncontrolled action of mine. Were they to be the parents of a brain-damaged child? Ok, a twenty-five-year-old woman but to them I would always be their child. Never before had I felt the need to put my arms around my mother and reassure her that everything would be all right. I could not be brain-damaged as I could hear and understand everything that they said to me and to each other.

I tried to slow down my rapid breathing. I suddenly realised that although there was a strong reaction with my right arm, my left one remained lifeless and heavy alongside my body under the duvet. This was the first time that the possibility that I could be paralysed entered into my head. Fortunately for me my body's reaction did not scare the staff as much as my family. One of the nurses turned smartly on her heels and left the room. She returned almost immediately with a large notepad and felttip pen in her hands and said: "Maybe you can write for us, Charlotte." She placed the pad on top of my bedding, and put the uncapped pen into my hand. My trembling right hand got an awkward grip on the pen. Something so familiar as writing felt so different to me. I had to concentrate hard to control the direction of the pen over the paper. In spite of the skewed direction, my small audience was able to read the message: *Call Granddad*.

My mother gave a reassuring squeeze to my arm and said, "Everything is going to be all right!" How could I explain to them that I was trapped inside this useless body?

I needed my granddad here with me. He would be able to tell them what I was going through. After having several heart attacks he knew how tremendously frustrating it was when your body let you down. I needed him to explain this especially to his daughter. I knew that he was old and physically weak, perhaps even unable to visit. I also knew that he would be able to offer my mum comfort and support. Note to my private checklist: Right arm was working; left, not!

9

Food and how to eat again

While I was lying in my hospital bed I had spent a lot of
time fantasising about food, whether it was something
that I had not eaten for some time or food that I had
never tried before. Until the pressure on my brain was
totally reduced and stabilised and my ability to speak
returned, I continued to write all of my requests on
the notepad. My first wish was for food and I wrote:
eat snow, which was a dish that my grandmother made
for me when I was a little girl. It was a porridge made
from rice flour and because of its white colour I always
called it snow. Obviously it would not be available on the
hospital menu but the nurse made a special request to
the kitchen staff. Luckily they were very happy to make
this dish for me. As soon as the nurse returned with the
steaming bowl of 'snow' my mother took the bowl and
sat on the edge of my bed. After letting it cool down for

a few moments she began to spoon-feed me. I reverted to my childhood and let her. The porridge was very nice but it would have been even better if they had sprinkled some more sugar and cinnamon on the top.

After only a few spoons the peace of the room was shattered when Vibsen and my brother, Peter, burst into the room.

"What the hell do you think you are doing, Mother?" my brother said. He always spoke as if he was still in the army issuing orders to subordinates in his regiment.

"Feeding my daughter. What does it look like, Peter?" my mother replied in a gentle voice. Before she even had time to refill the spoon Peter was taking it from her.

"Please leave the room. Charlotte is a grown woman and does not need your help with her food."

I watched my mother leave us without a murmur of protest. After the door closed behind her Peter placed the spoon into my right hand and the bowl in front of me on top of the duvet.

"Now, Charlotte, if you are to make a full recovery you must start by learning to feed yourself."

With a lot of concentration I managed to lift the spoon to where I believed my mouth was. After some time and a packet of wet wipes later I managed to work my way through the bowl of porridge.

My next request was when I felt very thirsty. I wrote on my notepad, *Coca-Cola*. This was one thing that my dad could do for me. He took off and went in search of a vending machine. Note to checklist: Eating and drinking skills. The next day I found myself in desperate need of ice cream and not just any ice cream; I wanted liquorice-flavoured ice cream. So Dad and Vibsen were off driving round to all of the shops in Aalborg in search of it for me. My next demand was much easier for them: grilled chicken and chips. Luckily for us there was a fast-food outlet opposite the hospital.

Slowly, as the pressure inside my brain reduced, my speech began to return to me. However, I was still having a few problems with words coming out back to front. In spite of the odd word, it was wonderful for me to be able to communicate verbally again, even if not everybody could understand what I tried to say. I put 'speech' on my checklist.

10

Jesper and Jens

Weeks had passed since my brain haemorrhage and my speech was slowly returning to normal. I asked the people who came to visit me, "Have you seen Jesper, the young man I was having dinner with the night I got sick?" I had no memory of him coming to see me in the hospital.

Nobody had mentioned his name. When I asked my parents and sister about him they obviously knew who he was, but my mother answered without delay, "Jesper is gone. Don't worry about him." I looked over at my dad and sister. They added nothing to Mum's comment but both looked away from me so that I could not catch their eye. It was not that I thought Jesper and I had a future together. I just wanted to see him and say thank you; maybe hear his version of our evening in the Greek restaurant.

It seemed to me that after my period in the coma my hearing had sharpened. From my bed I could easily follow conversations taking place in the corridor outside my room. One day my curiosity was piqued when I heard an unknown voice ask a nurse, "Where can I find Charlotte?"

"She is in room number seven just down the corridor."

A few seconds later an unknown pregnant woman in a nurse's uniform tapped on my door and entered. She smiled and said, "Hi, Charlotte. I am Helle. I am the wife of a friend of Jesper's. He's in Århus for a job interview. He'll visit you soon when he is back in Aalborg."

And she left as quickly as she had appeared.

Time passed slowly. I guessed it was afternoon now as the light through my window was less bright. There was a light tap on the door. In walked a doctor, his white coat flapping as he pushed a metal trolley in front of him. On the top of the trolley I could see a flipchart and several glasses of a red liquid. He looked very nice and he smiled as he spoke.

"Hello, Charlotte, I am Jens Haase, the surgeon who performed the operation on your brain. Charlotte, I have to tell you that you are a very lucky young woman. If it were not for the prompt action of the young man you were dining with calling for the ambulance, I would not be here having this conversation with you." I did not feel very lucky lying there but I managed to smile before he continued. "You suffered from a brain haemorrhage."

I gave him a new smile and asked, "Why did this happen to me?"

The doctor hesitated a bit before answering. "Now it gets a bit technical. First I will have to explain that arteries take oxygen and nutrition to the brain. Veins carry blood with less oxygen and waste products away from the brain back to the heart. You had what we doctors call an arteriovenous malformation or an AVM. When this occurs a tangle of blood vessels in the brain or on the surface of the brain bypasses normal brain tissue and directly diverts blood from arteries to veins. It means that brain tissue suffers from a lack of oxygen and nutrition. Many of these AVM are fragile and can burst and cause a bleeding, just as happened to you.

"It also happens to approximately one per hundred thousand people per year. More for men than women and mostly between the ages of twenty-five and fifty. The glasses with red liquid on my trolley are to show you how much blood we drained from your brain before starting to operate on you. Do you now understand how lucky you have been?" I nodded without a word. He smiled at me. "However, I am sorry because it is impossible for me to say if it was the sudden build up of pressure in your brain or something that happened during your operation that has caused you to be paralysed."

I looked up at the doctor and I saw the sorrow in his eyes. I tried to smile but I felt as if the muscles in my face had decided to work in their own way. It came across like a crooked grin. At least he knew I understood what he had told me.

I was paralysed.

Dr Jens Haase continued to speak and I tried to listen.

"Charlotte, I can't say exactly how good a physical recovery you will have. My assessment of you is that you are young, determined and strong. You should make a reasonable recovery. Also, we are treating you for epilepsy because as expected after the operation you had a couple of epileptic seizures."

Now I began to understand the seriousness of my situation and said to myself, *I am young, disabled and epileptic.*

11

That fateful night

As doctor Jens Haase said his goodbye and left still pushing his metal trolley, my family arrived again. My brother, Peter, was back. The doctor's words were still running through my brain and I could feel tears begin to form behind my closed eyelids. I was not alone and so would not give in to the much needed relief that flowing tears would bring me. As they all settled down around me I asked my mum, "Have you all been here since 12 April?" They all nodded but my mother answered, "Dad and I arrived shortly after midnight and Peter very soon after." She slowly contined to talk about that night.

"We sat for eight hours in the little waiting room outside the operating theatre," Peter added, with a huge smile on his face. "We were waiting outside the room where only people who can save lives may enter. Is that not what you said, Mother?"

She tried to ignore Peter and she looked at me before she continued. "I prayed for you, the doctors and nurses all the time you spent on the operating table and while we were waiting for you to come round after your operation." My family was not a particularly religious one but my mother was raised in a different way.

Then my father said to me, "I spent the time thinking of where we went wrong; what had we done that might have caused this tragedy?" I gave him a crooked smile hoping it conveyed all of the warmth and love I felt for him. I knew he found no solace in religion, only in rational explanations, and this, in his eyes, was neither rational nor had an explanation.

My sister then interrupted. "I am sorry. I came later because Tommy was away on a business trip. I couldn't leave the children alone in the house." I gave her a big, warm smile too.

Our mother, always the peacemaker, responded quickly. "The most important thing was that you came as soon as you could." Mum then continued to speak. "Marie had made a bottle of hot coffee which Peter brought and we drank it while waiting. At intervals during the night a nurse came to check on us and gave us a little information as to what was happening in the theatre."

My father interrupted with a smile on his lips, "When the operation was finished the Lord himself made an appearance."

Mum took over again. "He means that Dr Jens Haase came out to speak to us. We were all dozing a little when the door opened and the doctor was standing in the space with a glowing white light surrounding him."

Now Peter interrupted her saying, "I mostly saw blood on his surgical gown."

"He looked like a craftsman at the end of his working day," added my dad.

Peter replied, "He is a craftsman!"

Mum got up from the chair. "Jens Haase is a neurosurgeon, and one of the best in Denmark!" She now sounded very angry and raised her voice telling them, "He saved Charlotte's life." Dad and Peter gave her an apologetic look and lowered their eyes to the floor. So Mum took over again. "Later a nurse came out to explain to us that you were being taken down to the intensive care ward and that we would be able to see you in there. When we arrived you had been transferred from the stretcher to a normal ward bed. We got very scared when we saw your partly shaved head and all of the drainage tubes coming from your skull. You had various tubes in your arms. They were replacing lost blood. You had monitors that would activate the drugs that were necessary to help you recover. You also had a catheter attached to your bladder. But the worst thing was the wheezing of the respirator helping you breathe as it pumped oxygen round your battered body."

I could see the tears in her eyes. Unbeknownst to me, this had been a most traumatic and violent experience for her, for the whole family.

12

The visit

One morning, three weeks after my brain haemorrhage, a nurse came into my room.

"Hello, Charlotte. I'll be removing the catheter from your bladder."

I gave her a large smile and replied, "Oh, I am sorry as it has been my long-term and faithful companion." She got the humour,and smiled back at me.

"I am sorry but it is time to move on."

"Okay, but at least I will still have the wheelchair as the last visible evidence of how sick I have been."

A few days before, the nurses had started to make me sit for some hours in a big, heavy wheelchair with a support system to hold my head. The nurse laughed out loud. It had not been a pleasant experience to have a catheter. Luckily for me I was unconscious when it was inserted into my bladder. Now to have one removed was a painful situation, but I didn't have any choice.

I was so looking forward to being able to sit on a toilet and pee for myself. Unfortunately it was not as easy as I hoped it would be. After several hours and many repeated attempts I still failed to relax my bladder muscles enough to let nature take its course. Desperation began to show in both me and the nurses. They had tried everything to make my position a little more comfortable. They kept me going with plenty of fresh cold water and orange juice. They told me stories of being caught in heavy rain showers. One even told me about fountains and waterfalls, while they left the taps running for the sound effects. Nothing happened.

"Charlotte, we have decided to offer you an adult diaper."

I looked at her with wide, open eyes. "A diaper!"

"It is just in case your bladder muscles suddenly work at an inconvenient time."

To put on the diaper was one of the most humiliating experiences for me. Not only because it was an adult nappy but also because of the huge baggy underwear and shapeless sweatpants I had to wear to cover it up.

It was just my luck that this was also the moment that Jesper, my knight in shining armour, arrived. I immediately recognised his bright eyes, round cheeks and brown hair. He was wearing a smart white shirt, great jeans and a quilted down gilet.

Just the sight of him made my blood run hot and I could feel a blush come to my pallid cheeks. Tears came to my eyes just because I saw the man who helped to save my life. They were tears of joy and gratitude as I now had the chance to meet my rescuer again.

"Boy, some date you turned out to be!" were the first words he spoke. He looked at me, smiling so much. His mouth was one big curve and his eyes sparkled as he leaned over to kiss my cheek. I grabbed hold of his hand. I was so afraid that if I let go he would disappear. He used only one hand but managed to pull over a chair so he could sit next to my wheelchair.

I felt the blush returning to my cheeks. I could not help thinking that he might have been my Prince Charming on a white horse. Any feelings I had for him that night were now transformed into feelings of relief, gratitude and thankfulness. Judging by the chaste kiss he had just given me I decided that there were no romantic vibrations coming from him either. It did not matter. Right now I was just so happy to breathe naturally again. He broke the intensity of the moment. "Can I take you away from here?"

I smiled. "Oh, yes, please do," was my hasty reply.

Quickly he got up from his chair, he eased his hand from mine and started to wheel me out of the room in a hurry. As we passed the nurse at her work station I called out a cheerful, "See you later", as if leaving the hospital was the most natural thing for me to do.

Jesper kept on pushing my chair through the large vestibule of the hospital, out of the main entrance and across the parking lot. I began to think that he was going to kidnap me. He continued to walk me down the road to a crossing. We stopped even though the pedestrian light was green. We did not cross. Instead Jesper stopped and took of his gilet. He bent over and lifted my left, paralysed arm through the arm hole and pulled the down gilet round my other shoulder before helping me with my right arm. While he was doing this the traffic lights changed and the cars started to rush past us. It took a little while before the green man flashed again and it was safe for us to cross. I still had no idea where we could be going. When he slowed down to enter the city athletic stadium on the other side of the road I was still in a state of utter confusion and he was not giving me any clues. Suddenly I felt his mouth close to my right ear and heard him whisper, "Are you ready?"

Without knowing for what, I just nodded and replied, "Yes!" Before I could form a sentence to ask 'Ready for what?' he was off, running as fast as possible pushing my cumbersome hospital wheelchair around the 400-metre track. When we reached the winning line I took hold of my left hand with my right and not without some difficulty and a fair bit of pain I lifted them to the heavens in a victory salute. Jesper stopped the chair and walked round to the front. He kneeled down on the gravel and looked at me with a large smile. "Congratulations, Charlotte, now you can start the race to recovery because you know that you can win." Today, I knew, it was the start of my 'Dream Mile'.

On our return to my room we stopped by the vending machine and Jesper bought me a bottle of Cola Light and took one for himself.

He parked my wheelchair by a table in the vestibule and sat down on a chair opposite me. We clinked our bottles in salute raising a silent toast. I was bursting with curiosity and desperate to hear his version of what had happened at the Greek restaurant, how his job interview had gone and what his plans were for the future.

"I am sorry, Charlotte, 12 April is a bit blurred for me," he began. "All I can tell you is that you felt sick and so I called an ambulance." I could see he did not feel comfortable talking about it. So I did not pressure him. He continued, "I felt a little uncomfortable staying at the hospital with your family as they were in shock, so I left. The next day I returned to see how you were progressing. There, I met your boyfriend, Kristian. That meeting was a bit awkward so I decided not to return. I kept myself informed about you through a friend's wife, Helle, as she works at the hospital."

I took a sip of my Coke. "We hadn't done anything wrong, had we?" I asked him.

"No!" he replied laughing as he took my left hand in his. "You know that feeling of when you are driving and the police stop you for no reason; you panic and get a sweaty palm. That was how I felt around your family and Kristian."

I smiled. "Did you get the job in Århus?"

He seemed relieved when we changed the subject. He told me in detail about the interview, his new job and plans for the future. He let go of my hand and took out a business card from his wallet and gave it to me.

"This is from a hotel in Århus where I am working

for the time being. There is someone in the reception on duty twenty-four hours a day if you want to call me. Please!"

Jesper looked at me and as a natural development of our conversation he was expecting me to tell him how I was. Half of me felt as if we were just getting to know each other. The other half felt as if I had known him forever.

My head was full of words but all that came out was, "I can't pee!" A very confused Jesper looked at me as I slowly told him the story of the removal of the catheter, lots of drinking and running of taps as the nurses tried anything and everything. In the end and much to my surprise without any embarrassment I said: "I have to wear an adult diaper."

"Charlotte, please, you must telephone me as soon as you are able to pee again. Promise?" Stunned by Jesper's response I could only nod and agree to do so.

I continued to look at him sitting across from me while he drank his soda. Somehow he was still a stranger but one who so nearly could have become a new boyfriend. Now I knew that it would never happen and I was okay with it. Our conversation had been one of the best and most intimate I could recall since getting sick and I would have liked it to go on for much longer. Eventually he pushed me back into my room where we gave each other a warm hug of affection and said as one, "See you!" My eyes followed him through the open door as he walked away towards the lift. I watched as he raised his hand to press the call button. The lift arrived and as the doors opened he turned to wave. I smiled as the doors closed taking him away from me again. I continued to watch the digital numbers as they counted to the ground floor. I heaved a big sigh.

Alone again I put on my headphones.I played one of my favourite love songs written and sung by Lis Sørensen. It was only later when I took them off I realised that my cheek was wet. Despite a calm physical appearance, my inner self was broken-hearted. I cried for myself; tears of a possible love lost and maybe a little self-pity? I didn't know which but they cleansed me and I fell into a deep, refreshing sleep.

On his rounds the next day the doctor stopped and told me, "Charlotte, I am going to send you to visit our urologist to have an internal examination. We need to check out your bladder for any signs of a physical problem." I just nodded an acceptance.

A few days after his visit Jesper called me. I was watching the television in the common room so the nurse brought me the ward phone. It was fixed to a small trolley so the phone could be wheeled to a patient. Luckily for me I was the only person in the room as I had to tell him that in spite of many tries I could not pee properly. I was still wearing the diaper.

The miracle happened the next day. As always it was a busy morning. Just as the staff were rushing around distributing medication, making sure that we were bathed and dressed, I got the feeling of heat spreading between my legs. It felt warm, wet and very unpleasant. First, my brain told me how disgusting it was for a grown woman to pee in her pants. Then a feeling of relief took over. My bladder was working at last. Now I had to learn how to have some control over it. Very soon the warmth of the liquid turned cold and my pants were wet and uncomfortable. I tugged on the string next to my bed to call one of the duty nurses. Despite it being a busy time of day, a nurse came quickly to see me. Normally I would have no problem with a male nurse but this male nurse was different. The male nurse, Palle, came from my home town. In fact, he was only two classes above me in school.

"I am so sorry, Palle, but I really need to have a female nurse, please."

I was so embarrassed that I might offend him but he just said, "Of course, Charlotte. I will find one for you."

Within a few minutes a female nurse came. "Congratulations, Charlotte, things are getting back to normal at last." Her congratulations reminded me to make a mental note to add peeing to my checklist.

Once I was washed and changed I wheeled myself to the payphone to call Jesper. The pleasant-sounding receptionist answered: "I am sorry. He is in a meeting and cannot be disturbed." During the course of the next few hours I made more calls and spoke to a now very irritated woman who said, "I have left a number of messages for him but he is obviously too busy to call."

I apologised to her and asked, "Can you please leave one more message? Just write:*Charlotte can pee!*"

Later that day a huge bouquet of flowers arrived for me with the attached card reading *Congratulations on peeing.* It was not until much later the same evening that Jesper could phone me to congratulate me. Even though I was so happy to receive the bouquet from him, I felt rather depressed that I, a twenty-five-year-old woman, received flowers for being able to pee. It was a sobering thought that this might be a sign of my future – a future bereft of passionate kisses from a hot man. A lump of lead filled my stomach. It was a lump of pent-up frustration and anger over why the bleeding happened in my brain and not someone who was intent on destroying their own life with drugs or alcohol. I didn't deserve this.

13

My sunshine

I was not exactly in the best of moods when Lotte unexpectedly walked into my room. She said to me the same thing as everyone else who came to visit: "It is wonderful to see you sitting up in the wheelchair." Her face dropped as I looked at her through my half-closed eyes.

"Lotte, tell me exactly what you see when you look at me? How do I really look? I need you to tell me the truth, please." Poor Lotte. I knew it was impossible for her to lie to me. Instead of an answer she turned round and left the room, only to return a few minutes later with a hand mirror borrowed from one of the nurses.

It was shocking to see myself in the small mirror. I could feel my throat begin to tighten and tears form in my eyes. The right side of my scalp had been completely shaved and was covered by a gauze patch which protected the scar from my recent operation. It started from the upper part of my forehead and it ran all the way back down to my neck. My face was very pale and the left side was clearly frozen. When I tried to smile only the right side of my lips moved upwards. There was a small stream of drool running from the left corner of my mouth. If it were not for my open, clear green eyes you could mistake me for a corpse. Luckily for me the hair on my right side was still thick and flame- coloured although it was flat and lifeless. It needed a good wash but still it reminded me of how I once looked and hopefully would look again.

There had been many opportunities for me to look in the mirror before. I could have asked a nurse for one, or just looked in the bathroom mirror while the nurse helped me bathe. Up until now it had not been a priority for me. I had needed to keep all my energy and thoughts on reclaiming my life and regaining control of my body and brain rather than worring about how I looked. At least that was what I thought. I looked back to Lotte and said with a tearful voice, "I am like a corpse!"

Her only reply was a phrase that we used so many times at school: "Life is a bitch and then you die."

I tried to smile in response. "But I am not dead! I just look like I am. I need to start to look like a living person again."

She nodded. "Okay, you may not look the same as before but at least we can try to improve what we have left."

Lotte was a woman who never travelled light. She

always carried with her a huge, seemingly bottomless bag. She dug down deep and eventually pulled out a small red leather case, a hairbrush and lastly an elasticated hairband. She then proceeded to brush my remaining hair into a ponytail that sat on the top of my head like a fountain. I looked into the mirror and I gave a crooked smile of some relief as I could see a small resemblance to my old self.

Rummaging in the red leather case she brought out a manicure set and reached out to take my left, paralysed hand. As she touched my hand it immediately cramped. "I am sorry, Lotte, this hand has a will of its own. You will have to use some muscles here."

She now gripped my hand with both of hers and tried to stretch my fingers. "Tell me if it hurts." It didn't not hurt and I didn't tell her that it felt a bit intimate to have another person touching the paralysed part of my body. She decided to do one finger at a time and slowly she managed to give me a manicure. Then she went to my bathroom and returned with a warm, wet flannel. She proceeded to wash my face. After that she moved behind my chair and began to massage my face with one of her creams. Slowly, I felt human again. Finally, she pulled out a mascara from her bag and started to put some on my eyelashes. Her face was so close to mine that I could feel her breath. Even though she was my best friend, it felt uncomfortable for me. Lotte doing my make-up woke up a voice inside me. I heard a voice in my head. *Come on, Charlotte. Get back into the battlefield. You do not want other people to decide how you should look!* I tried to ignore the voice but realised it was my own inner will. I knew it was as stubborn as me so even though I enjoyed what Lotte was doing I said, "Thank you, Lotte. It has helped a lot but please stop."

After Lotte left I picked up the mirror and took a long look at myself. I did not think that I was attractive, but for the first time since I arrived in the hospital I felt alive again. It was at that moment I decided I was going to hold on to life for as long as I could. I was now filled with a new and more positive feeling of hope. I was determined to push out all of the anger and frustration that I had been holding on to. My new look did not go unnoticed by the hospital staff and from that moment I became known as the cheeky young woman with a ponytail; which was so much better than being the disabled woman in room number seven.

I was still feeling good about myself when a couple of hours later Kristian turned up. Up until that day his visits had only coincided with other people's and our conversations had always been about practical matters such as the packing up and storage of belongings from my flat. It was on the first floor and so it would not be possible in the near future for me to return because of the steep stairs. Besides, the apartment only had a bathtub and no shower. Sometimes we chatted about how his studies were progressing but never about us.

As he walked into my room that day there was a look of surprise on his face. He saw me with brushed hair, a little make-up and manicured nails. For the first time I felt we were looking at each other as the equal adults we were and as the lovers we used to be.

He pulled up a chair and sat next to me. He turned to look into my eyes. He took a deep breath and just came right out with, "Charlotte, you know that my birth sign is Leo and we lions will not accept infidelity in a partner!"

I wanted to protest but I was too stunned by this comment. It was so absurd. For a second I considered an appeal to his better nature, that he was mistaken, but I could see by the look on his face it would be pointless and deep down I understood that our relationship was over. I just let him continue with his prepared speech.

"Charlotte, I have finished packing your belongings from the flat and have put them in storage in the basement of your school. The head has given approval for this. Your stuff will be kept safe for you for as long as necessary. My brother will be there tomorrow with a trailer to collect my remaining property." At this point I just wished he would get up and leave me alone. It turned out he had decided to prolong the agony by staying. We talked about everything but ourselves. It was much to my relief that Tine and Jens arrived for a visit. Kristian quickly said his goodbye and left. That night was long and sleepless and, for once, the love songs of Lis Sørensen were of no help to me.

The next morning, after my usual breakfast in bed, a nurse came to help me take a shower and get dressed. My daily routine was still that after I was dressed I would spend the day sitting in my wheelchair. I could see the spring sunshine through the windows and I decided to wear a lighter pair of sweatpants and a striped T-shirt. I felt that it would do me good to leave my room and sit in the fresh air for a change. My now ex-lover Kristian arrived and I asked, "Can you please take me outside?"

He gave me a fatherly look. "It is too cold for you sitting still in the wheelchair."

His concern made me smile. "I will wear an extra sweater."

"Okay then, but I am in a bit of a hurry as my brother is coming with the car and trailer."

I told Kristian to take me to the small corner left of the main entrance where I could be sheltered from the cool breeze. He left me and went to find a secure parking space for his brother's car and trailer.

The sun's warm rays caressed my pale face. Soon I had to use my right arm to shield my eyes from its brightness. It was a small price to pay to feel the rays of pure energy working their way into my tired body. All too soon Kristian was back. He stood in front of me. He was talking continuously but I was not taking any notice of him or of what he said. I just could not understand why he bothered to come back for a final visit. I picked up some of the phrases he used such as: 'Not the woman I fell in love with' and 'I leave for practical reasons.'

I had had enough of him. In a loud voice I interrupted him. "Go away, you are blocking my sunshine!" He stepped sideways and stood there in uncomfortable silence. We both knew that it was over and that there was nothing left for us to say to each other. So I just told him to wheel me back into my room. On our arrival we looked at each other. Then he bent over to give me a farewell kiss. I turned my face away from him only to feel a light brush of his lips on my cheek. I didn't turn back to see him walk away. For the rest of the day I was full of mixed emotions. My dream of a boyfriend, lover, husband and a family of my own was lost. I was, of course, sorry about our break-up and the fact that he was not there when I needed him most. I also felt relieved that he was gone even though my life was in chaos.

I had been to hell. The man who I thought loved me had dumped me. I was on my own and in my new life. This life of mine was going to be under my control; I knew that I would have to fight for myself. My mixed feelings of relief and disappointment sat heavy on my chest and I had to talk to someone. I tried to talk to my nurses but they did not really understand what I was going through. They were very kind to me. One nurse even telephoned my parents to let them know what had happened. My mother wanted to speak to me. "My dear Charlotte, I am really disappointed in him. How could he let you down during the most difficult time of your life? He should be standing by you and supporting you. Not running away."

I interrupted her. "Mum, it's okay. Let's not talk more about it right now!" "Sure, darling." I hung up.

I might have been sad and disappointed and totally let down by Kristian but that night I slept like a baby…

14

Changes

A sunny morning, 1 June. It had been more than five weeks since I woke up from my coma. When my parents arrived that morning I told them, "We need to go into town today. I am in desperate need of some new clothes before I am transferred to the new hospital." I was to be transferred to a paraplegic rehabilitation unit at the hospital in Viborg. The rehabilitation unit was primarily for people suffering from spinal cord injury but they also tried to help rehabilitate hemiplegic patients such as me. My dad looked at me.

"Okay. When?"

I gave him a look as if I did not understand anything and answered in an unpleasant tone. "Now, of course!"

My parents looked at each other and I just knew my bad temper made them think that I was changed as a person. I could see the fear in my mother's eyes. They both replied. "Sure!"

On our way into town I breathed in the city life with my mouth wide open. I heard the noise of the traffic as people rushed about, everyone caught up with their own busy lives. I observed everything that was going on around me as if I was seeing things for the first time. Even Dad's complaints about the wonky wheel on the hospital wheelchair were music to my ears after the relative silence of the hospital. The feeling of the warm, early summer sun as it touched my pale face filled me with new energy. I said nothing when Dad pushed my chair into the entrance of Salling, the department store in Aalborg. I was almost overwhelmed to be back in the shop I had so often visited whilst attending teacher training college. The shop seemed so much bigger from my place in the wheelchair. Quickly I scanned the ground floor looking for anyone that I might know. I was not ready to be recognised sitting in the chair with a large scar on one side of my head and a funny hairstyle on the other. Suddenly I realised that I had no money with me. "We have to go to a cash machine."

Mum leant over to tell me, "Your brother has spoken with your bank and explained to them your situation and the need to get your finances in order. We will pay for what you need to buy."

I felt so furious with him. How dare he take control of my finances without my permission. My blood was boiling through my ravaged body. I did not need anyone to take over my life. I wanted to scream out at the injustice of it. Maybe my mother could see what was happening to me? She put her hand on my shoulder to calm me down. The sensible side of my brain then moved into action and I remembered that for the last two months I had been unable to go to the bank myself. Of course, my brother had done what he thought was best for me. I could not understand why he did not think to talk to me about it. It was not as if I could not hear, speak or understand him. I could feel myself becoming legally incapacitated and it made me furious.

We made it to the first floor of the shop. I was lucky to see a pair of jeans with an elasticated waistband that I wanted to try on. After two months in a hospital bed my body shape had changed so much and not just because I was partially paralysed. I was scared. Originally I had been fed through tubes inserted directly into my stomach. When they were removed I started to eat only my favourite foods and that combined with the lack of exercise had caused my body to now have extra stomach fat. I would need to increase the size of my jeans. I had gone from a size small to large in one go. I also needed to be able to pull them on without undoing the zip or buttons. With one hand that would be difficult for me. I wheeled myself into a narrow fitting room and closed the curtains. There I managed to take off the hated ugly sweatpants and with a lot of difficulty put on the new jeans. The next thing I knew my mother came in without my asking. She swished open the curtains and tried to pull up the jeans for me. Although we were alone in the fitting room, I felt exposed and embarrassed by her actions. I managed to bite my tongue and say nothing. From there we went into the underwear and lingerie department. My mother found a pair of knickers and a white top with green polka dots. She handed them over to me. She said, in what for me seemed to be a very loud voice, "Charlotte, these are perfect for you as you can't open and close a bra with only one hand."

This time I replied to her. I almost shouted. "That may be true! But I am a grown woman. I wear underwired bras. I am not your twelve-year-old daughter buying my first bra!"

I hated the changes to my body and my mother's comments. I was still seething as we left the store with my new jeans and the green spotted underwear in a bag. I was angry because my mother was right. I was not able to open and close my own bra. I decided that in future, when I could decide, it was going to be my choice and my choice only. Back at the hospital I was still angry, or maybe mostly sad. I only wanted to be alone so I said, "Please leave. I want to be alone!" Luckily my parents did not ask permission to stay. They left without a word.

For almost two hours I sat alone in my room just staring out of the window. My brain was working overtime and my emotions were somersaulting between irritation and anger, humiliation and frustration – all of those negative emotions. Finally, I decided that it was not me who needed to change. It was the people surrounding me. They needed to alter their perception of me. They were the ones who had to realise that I was an independent twenty-five-year-old woman with a medical condition and not a helpless cripple in need of their sympathy. I had to restore my old self; get back to who I was, to the old Charlotte who never gave up the fight. I certainly knew where and how to start.

I wheeled myself out of my room and made my way back down the corridor towards the intensive care unit. I wanted to speak to the two nurses who had taken care of me and I hoped they were working that night. As I got closer I could hear them talking. The one with the loudest voice was clearest.. The second, with the hoarse voice, was a little more indistinct. I could make out that some tubes needed replacing. I knew one of them had to come out to get the tubes, so I sat in my chair and waited patiently for one to come out.

In my head I had prepared what I was going to say but when the doors suddenly opened the carefully chosen words fled from my brain. So, I was not the first to speak.

"Sorry, you are not allowed in here," said the nurse, without looking at me. I made no reply and she looked down at me. "I am sorry, Charlotte. I didn't recognise you."

I knew I had to say what I had come here for; quickly, before she started the small talk. Just seeing her made me feel the same anger and frustration building up inside me as when I had been lying in intensive care. I clearly remembered how I had been stuck in my bed listening to the nurses talk about me, as if I were not there. I now looked directly at the nurse and I opened my mouth to speak. The voice that came out was flat and monotonous.

"Did you really think that I was so stupid to believe the crushed pills on my yogurt were muesli? Or did you think that I was just brain-damaged and wouldn't know the difference?"

In spite of my inner anger my voice sounded as if I were a TV presenter discussing boring fishing quotas. There was no variation in tone or cadence. It was just flat and all this did was to increase my sense of frustration.

I, of course, remembered that the doctor had explained this to me; that due to the pressure of the bleeding in my brain I could temporarily be suffering from what the medical world called aprosodia. It was also known as the inability to express emotions in language. The nurse put her hand on my left arm and pushed open the door. In a softer voice she called to her colleague. The hand touching my paralysed arm felt so patronising. I wanted to pull away from her, if only I could.

The other nurse came to the door without leaving the room. She looked back over her shoulder at the patients lying in their beds. Finally, she looked down at me and recognising me, said, "Hey, Charlotte, you are looking good."

I ignored her. I just repeated the words I'd used before, regarding the crushed pills. This time, to make sure that they understood what I felt, I almost shouted them. They gave each other a quick, frightened look. I continued in a slightly quieter voice. "You really need to get it sorted out who you want. Is it the one in the lift or the one you already have at home?" I could feel my confidence growing as I looked down at her legs. "I see that you have shaved your legs again. Which one is it for this time?" I turned my wheelchair around. I tried to suppress a giggle but failed miserably.

She replied, "Oh my God, did you hear me say that as well?" Although I felt happier because I had spoken out, I could feel a lump in my throat and tears falling from my eyes. I turned my chair a sharp left into the nearest toilet. There, I broke down with a loud sob. For the first time I let go and cried for the sorrow overwhelming my broken body. I felt dejected because I was afraid for my future. How could I ever get people to listen to me? What if I would always have such a boring, flat voice? How could people tell if I was angry or happy when I spoke to them? What if it turned out that I did have some permanent brain damage?

15

My future

Early the next morning I had an appointment with Dr Jens Haase in his office for a final check-up before being transferred to another hospital. After testing for reflex reactions he gave me the good news.

"Charlotte, although your body is working well neurologically, you will for a period need to continue to take the medicine to control your epilepsy."

I looked at him. "Lucky me!"

Once the physical examination was completed he said: "Maybe you might consider applying for a disability pension."

I just glared at him. "Dr Haase, I have no intention of claiming for a disability pension. I do have every intention of returning to work as soon as it is possible for me to do so."

Later that same day, returning to my room, I was

surprised to find the head teacher from my school waiting for me. I knew how busy he and the other teachers would be as this was the last day before school broke up for the long summer holidays. This was not the first time that he had visited. Before, I was not capable of even thinking about returning to work, let alone talking about it. I offered him a coffee and took a glass of cold water from the fridge for me. He looked around the room.

"I hear that you are leaving town?"

"Just for a short time. I am being transferred to the rehabilitation department in Viborg. I will be back for work in time for the children's return at the end of August."

As usual, his glasses had slipped down to the end of his nose. He looked over the frame and he said: "Good, I will expect you then." It seemed to me, he was the only person who saw what I was capable of, who believed that I was able to handle any challenge I faced. For a while we talked about what needed to be done before the school closed down for the holidays. "Goodbye, Charlotte. I am looking forward to seeing you back at work." He left me sitting in my wheelchair with a huge, lopsided grin on my face.

It was midsummer, eight weeks since I had woken up from my coma. It was always a very busy time in the restaurant and my mother was working, so that evening my father came to visit me alone. This time he brought in dinner for us both; fried chicken and French fries from the diner in front of the hospital. We sat together in the TV room eating our meal as I told him about my visit from the head teacher and our conversation. My father listened in silence and took his time before he responded.

"We need to see if you are able to walk again before you can even think about returning to work."

Disappointed by his response I snapped back at him, "Can you have some faith in my abilities? I know I will walk again."

I know that I was being unfair to him. I wanted him, I needed him, to encourage and push me to try harder.

Next morning he telephoned me. "Charlotte, if you are walking by the beginning of August I will pay for you, Mum and me to travel to France and visit your sister." I had, of course, visited my sister before I had my brain haemorrhage, but this chance to return to her beautiful home in the Sologne Forest gave me an added reason to get back on my own two feet. It would be a perfect holiday. She would be the perfect hostess. She would spoil us with fantastic food and wine, but what I would really enjoy about this trip was that my father would have to dig deep into his wallet to pay for it. He has always preferred to hide his money under his mattress than to spend it. This was going to be his way of motivating me to get up off my backside and get walking again.

16

Rehabilitation and repetition

I arrived at the rehabilitation unit on a Monday morning after being driven there by a patient transport car. The driver pushed the heavy monster that was my wheelchair and folded it to fit into the boot. On our arrival the chair was taken away and replaced by a smaller, lighter red chair (at last I now had my Ferarri coloured chair, the car of my dreams). This new chair was easier for me to handle using only my right hand.

The rehabilitation centre building and gardens were soaked with the hot July sunshine. The department consisted of two yellow single-storey buildings connected by a glass passage. It was situated near a beautiful lake. It didn't feel or look like a hospital but more like a small, private holiday camp or hotel. The nurse at the reception desk explained to me the theory behind this rehabilition centre. It was to return the client (we were not referred to as patients) to a near normal life. Because of this theory, they believed that the client would recover better if they were in control of their days. This meant the daily structure was loose. The only commitment was that we had to be present in the gymnasium when the physiotherapy sessions were booked for us. My room was a twin one and I was to share with another female patient. She was only there between therapy sessions and to sleep at night. The nurse gave me my weekly schedule telling me the times I was required to attend with my occupational therapist an examination by a neuropsychologist. After that I was on my own. For the first time since I was taken ill, I could feel that these professional people surrounding me saw me as a future independent adult and not just as a patient they had to look after. All I needed now was for my parents to see this and behave in the same way.

It was only a couple of hours after I arrived that I had my first scheduled appointment with Dorte, my physiotherapist. She made me feel so comfortable. She was a practical woman who understood my need to get on my own two feet and walk, even though, as she explained, "Charlotte, you will be crawling before walking again." The dark cloud of depression was descending on me again. Could it be true? I was only going to go backwards and not forwards. As we began our first session Dorte pulled a transparent sleeve over my paralysed arm. Once she had inflated this she said, "This will stabilise your paralysed arm, so you will be in a position that will enable you to balance and learn to crawl again." Dorte told me this as she helped me from my wheelchair and onto a large platform consisting of eight benches covered in leather pushed together.

It was with great difficulty that I managed to get up on to my knees and with Dorte's help put both of my hands palm down in front of me. I needed her help in manoeuvring my rigid left arm. Eventually, I was in position. Dorte then placed her hand on top of mine. I felt the heat passing from her hand into mine and with just a light touch I relaxed into this new experience. For the first time since 12 April I was down on all fours and feeling good. I lifted my head up and looked forward. I heard myself saying "Oh my God". It was if the words came out through my body and not my mouth, emanating from somewhere deep inside me. I did not know if it was because I could see the beautiful view of the sun dancing across the lake through the large picture windows, or if it was because I was back on all fours again. Dorte was certain that my surprise was because I was back to crawling on my hands and knees. She gave my stiff body a hug.

"Yes, it is a big thing. Please stay still to get your balance." We waited for a few minutes. I was concentrating so much, I forgot to breathe. When I eventually moved my right hand and leg forward there was a mighty 'thud' as I keeled over and collapsed onto my left side. My brain was telling my left arm and leg to hold me up but somehow the message was not getting through. Here I was, lying flat on my back with my left arm still sticking up into the air. I felt as if I was a young turtle that had been washed ashore and landed on its shell. It was a very embarrassing and degrading position to be in and I felt like crying. I was so upset with my failure to do such a simple manoeuvre. At least it made me realise just how far I had to go; how much work I needed to do to get back on my own two feet, not to mention an all-expenses-paid holiday in France.

Just after my third physiotherapy session my parents came to visit me. They had both taken the day off work. The weather forecast for the coming days was good, so I had asked Mum to bring me some shorts. I immediately changed into them. It was such a relief to be rid of those awful sweatpants. We had no particular plans of how to spend the day, so I asked them to take me into town. I felt another change coming on. On our arrival I looked around for a hairdresser. It was time to have my lopsided ponytail cut off and my remaining hair trimmed into a more adult style. Back at the centre in the afternoon with my new hairdo, I went for my second physio session of the day with Dorte. She smiled. "At last you are beginning to look like a woman again."

The first week passed by quickly. Between physiotherapy sessions I wheeled myself around talking to some of the other patients. Once, I was out on the terrace and met up with another young woman in a wheelchair. I thought her to be be about the same age as me, so I wanted to get to know her.

"Hello, I'm Charlotte. I'm twenty-five years old. How old are you?"

She stopped her wheelchair next to mine. "My name is Lise and I'm a year older."

I smiled at her to show I was happy to meet someone my age. "I'm from Aalborg and I work as a teacher."

"I live in Esbjerg, where I was working in a bank."

I smiled again. "Like me, you were lucky enough to be offered a place here." She looked at me with a surprised face. "Lucky or unlucky? It is hard work. I have given up with the physiotherapy. I do still attend the sessions but I am not trying very hard."

Now I looked surprised and I could not help it. My mouth moved before my brain. "Why? Don't you want to walk again?"

She looked at me as if my question came as a big surprise. She lit up a cigarette before answering me. "I think it will be easier to get a pension if I am still in a wheelchair."

Now I was in total shock. "I just can't believe that you would rather have a pension than be able to walk and work again!"

I said my goodbye and wheeled away. That, I have to say, was our first and last conversation.

I enjoyed every session I spent with Dorte and worked diligently to try to convince the muscles on the left side of my body to behave and to work as they were supposed to do. Maybe, if truth be told, Dorte was working even harder trying to loosen my tight muscles. I just lay there, while she pulled and pushed my very reluctant body. After three or four days, my impatience was beginning to show. I kept on complaining and telling her what I wanted to do when I could walk again. Dorte just kept working on me. She was so patient; oh, so patient with me. Dorte was a tall, strongly built woman. She had a warm, empathic personality and a soft, gentle look in her eyes. She was a woman who not only had the energy to love and look after her own children and family but she gave freely of her love to take care of us, her clients. She was, in my mind, truly the Danish version of Mother Theresa.

When I was not exercising, I spent my time dressed in shorts and a sun top sitting out on the large terrace by the lake. My skin was slowly changing from a pasty white to a soft golden colour. Just sitting out in the sun helped my spastic muscles relax. It was pure energy for body and soul. By the end of our first week I could kneel and shuffle forwards a little. When our time ended for the day, I received a slap on my bum from Dorte.

"A will of iron and a bum of steel, Charlotte. We are going to have you up and walking again."

"When?" I whispered in reply.

17

Magic

The first weekend was coming up and on the Friday, Lotte arrived to collect me. We had planned to spend my first weekend out of the hospital at her apartment in Århus. As soon as she saw me she stopped and said, "Oh my God, I thought it was a man in here! If you must have a man's haircut you could at least wear some mascara and try to look like a woman."

I looked up. "We will have to stop off on the way so that I can buy some," was the only response I could think of. As usual she was being honest with me, which was one of the things that I always liked about her. In the end we drove straight to her house and I decided to buy some mascara the next day. After a pleasant evening I felt a little tired so I went to bed early. It was so good to be out of the rehabilitation unit and in a normal environment for a change.

Saturday morning came and we decided to go shopping in the Magasin department store to buy some mascara and other odds and ends that I needed. Before we had even parked the car, however, I felt the pressure building up in my bladder. I still had less control of my bladder muscles than before so I was always happy to take the chance for an extra toilet stop. Lotte helped me get quickly into my wheelchair and we were soon speeding to the nearest staff member to ask for directions. I was trying to stop the store's sales girl we found from spraying me with her sample bottle of 'Magic Noir' while Lotte asked her for directions to the nearest toilets for the disabled. The very young shop assistant immediately pointed towards the rear of the shop. She was either wanting us away from her beautiful display of black and gold, or she saw the desperation in my eyes. Before I even managed to thank her I was being whisked through displays of leather handbags, gloves and suitcases towards the rear of the store and the safety of the toilets. With my good right hand I hung on tight to my seat. I was not sure if it was because of my precarious situation or the speed at which I was being propelled across the floor, but I felt so dizzy.

Suddenly, from behind a large display of handmade chocolates, there appeared a pushchair with a sleeping baby in front of me. A collision was imminent. I closed my eyes and prayed. If it were not for the quick reaction by both the mother and Lotte, baby and I would have shot out of our respective chairs and been flung across the marble floor. This time I managed a rushed apology before heading towards the toilet again. We arrived without further incident and Lotte grabbed the handle to pull open the door only to discover that it was locked with a notice pinned to the door saying: 'Please collect the key from the information desk'.

We both looked back in panic. The information desk was next to the 'Magic Noir' perfume stand. Now I was getting into a dangerous situation and needed to bring my right leg up to cross over my left to try to give some assistance to my poor bladder muscles. Lotte said quickly, "Probably best if I just run and get the key." For the first time since our arrival at the store she let go of the wheelchair handle and ran back to the information desk. I could see her hands flying all over the place as she asked them for the key. I lifted my right arm but it was no good. They could not see me behind the pile of chocolates. Lotte hastened back to me, her face contorted with laughter when she asked, "Which hand do you want?"

Now I was a bit desperate. "The one behind your back. Hurry up!" I answered with water in my eyes. Lotte brought her hidden hand to the front so that I could see what she was holding. The key looked more like a weapon taken from the Middle Ages. It was enormous. It should have had a key tag attached with a label saying 'You'd better not be disabled to use this key'!

Giggling hysterically she passed over the key to me. It was so very heavy and the grotesqueness of the situation we were in was making me laugh as well. I stopped myself in time before I lost it completely and peed in my jeans. Too late. I could feel a trickle of pee leaking from my body. Lotte slammed open the door and shoved me inside. Her tone was as if she was talking to a dog. "Stay!" she said to me. "I will go and buy some clean panties for you." Left alone in the toilet and with great difficulty I managed to take off my wet clothing before washing myself and the wet patch on my jeans. I dried them with the electric hand dryer on the wall. I sat there, bare bum in front of the large mirror in my Ferarri red wheelchair, short hair and no mascara. I desperately could do with a miracle or at least a quick spray from the 'Magic Noir' woman. I only had a few minutes for self-pity before Lotte returned with my new panties. This time, not boring white with green spots. These were black cotton edged with white lace. At least I might feel a little bit sexier in them even if I didn't look it. Along with the panties Lotte had bought me some mascara and so, still giggling like a pair of schoolgirls, we repaired our make-up. We made our way back to the information desk to return the weapon and had a quick spray of perfume.

By now we were both in need of a drink and so I was pushed to a nearby café. I was so grateful that I had Lotte to take me out into the real world.

"It is so inconvenient having to use the wheelchair all the time," I said to Lotte while sitting in the café.

"I agree. It's time you get out of it, then," she answered me.

"That, my dearest Lotte, is exactly what I am working on."

18

Up and go

Back in the rehabilitation unit after my weekend of freedom I knew that I would be having a busy week ahead. I had physiotherapy with Dorte every day to strengthen my muscles. It was now Wednesday of my second week and my morning session was with Dorte. As usual she started by saying, "Wheel over to the leather couches. "But I did not move. I stayed silent and still in the middle of the room not looking at anything but my hands sitting in my lap. Dorte picked up her chair and placed it down in front of me and looked at me. Still without looking up I said to her: "This doesn't work for me, the wheelchair I mean. I want to walk. No, I need to walk so that I can start putting my life together and return to work at the end of the school summer holidays. I promised them that I would be back by then. Furthermore, my stingy father promised me an all-expenses-paid trip to France if I could walk by 1 August."

We sat in silence for a few moments before Dorte said: "Right. Wheel yourself over to the parallel bars then."

Quickly, I manoeuvred myself to the bars, got in between the two upright supports and grabbed the bar on the right. I didn't understand what was happening. As soon as I started to pull myself from the chair with my stronger hand the left side of my body responded by becoming extremely spastic. My left arm cramped up and came towards my face. My left foot turned making it impossible for me to place it down on the floor. But that was not the end. I had forgotten to lock the wheels of my chair. It now shot away from under me so that I could not sit down. All I could do now was to heave my trembling body over the bar. There I hung like the weekly washing until I felt my chair safely back under me. I was sitting there feeling both embarrassed and humiliated. Without hesitation, Dorte put her arm round me and said, "Nice try. We can come back to them later. Let's have a rest for the moment."

I wheeled myself out of the gymnasium, onto the terrace and into my little corner where the angle of the wall sheltered me from the breeze and the sun warmed my body. Across the lake I could see the sports hall where less than a year ago I had spent a long weekend on a training course for teachers and we spent hours playing volleyball. *Shit! Now I am back in this bloody wheelchair and I will never play it or any other ball game again!* My head was spinning. What went wrong? I had been walking for nearly twenty-four years and now I couldn't even pull myself up and stand. For the time being I had to swallow my pride and accept defeat. It was hurting me so much. My head was so full of thoughts of failure that tears followed quickly and soon they were pouring down my cheeks. I could hear footsteps coming up behind me and so I quickly rubbed my face to dry them with the back of my right hand; of course my left hand was not working. I could feel self-pity coursing through my veins again. "Stop being so hard on yourself! I understand that this is a difficult time for you but give us some time and we will help you back on your feet again. "Now I saw Lasse, one of the other physiotherapists, standing next to me. All I could do was turn my face away from him. "Charlotte, please just listen to me. I know that you don't understand why it is suddenly so difficult to do something as basic as walking. I can understand some of the frustration you are feeling now."

Turning my head to face him I replied, "A child of two can start to walk when it decides it doesn't want to crawl any more." I looked him in the eyes.

"My point exactly, Charlotte. From what I hear, you don't want to crawl any more either!"

Later that afternoon Dorte was back and she told me to wheel myself into one of the conference rooms. I spoke first: "I know you want to tell me that it is okay to be angry and to get frustrated – but, you don't need to. Really, I do not want to talk about it. I know that it is something that I need to get over in my own way."

Dorte gave me a big smile. "You are wrong. This is not a talk about feelings and emotions," she replied.

Dorte used a large picture book and a plastic model of a human skeleton to explain in great detail how the body worked to send messages from the brain via electric pulses to our muscles. This was just what I remembered from biology classes at school. She was sounding like one of my former teachers and she kept repeating to me: "Let go in the hip, swing the lower leg forward until the heel touches the floor, then put your weight on it and roll forwards on the foot until you reach the tip of your toes." Then we both repeated this several times before she told me to wheel myself into the gym.

Instead of going back to the bars she told me to wheel myself over to the massage table. There, she systematically massaged all of my muscle from my neck down to the toes spending more time on the left side of my body. When I felt heavy and relaxed she told me that it was time to return to that morning's crime scene. I wheeled myself back to the parallel bars, this time with the wheels safely locked. Dorte knelt in front of me and placed both of my feet onto the floor and told me to stand up as slowly as possible.It seemed to take forever but eventually I was standing between the two bars. Dorte then told me to repeat the words we spoke earlier. As I said them, I was to put them into practice. The hip part was easy, but as I could not control my left leg when I swung it forward, I had difficulty in placing the heel on the floor. Dorte leaned forward and took my left leg in her hands. She gently controlled my movement and put my heel onto the floor. Slowly I moved to put all of my weight onto my left leg. I was now in a position to lift my right leg and take my first small, insecure step. I could not say that it was a great or even a beautiful movement. I could not manage the part where I rolled from the heel to the toe; it was more of a stiff wooden leg making the step. At least my effort made Dorte laugh and she gave me a round of applause.

"It may not be a ten for artistic merit, Charlotte, but you definitely get a ten for trying," she said in between breaths

19

Girls on tour

In spite of my earlier objections to Lotte's plan for a trip to Skagen, which is the most northern town in Denmark, I was quite happy that by my third Friday afternoon in the rehabilitation unit I was sitting in the passenger seat of her little, old Fiat. To know that we had several hours of driving ahead of us before we would arrive at our destination made me feel comfortable. I was physically exhausted after a full week of hard exercise on the parallel bars. So I was too tired to say anything when, with a huge grin on her face, she paraphrased the Duran Duran song by singing 'Girls on tour, Girls on tour'. I was almost asleep even before we had left Viborg.

Lotte had insisted that we make this trip. She ignored any protest.

"Maybe it is better for me to stay and keep on doing my exercises?"

"Come on, Charlotte. We always used to go to Skagen during our summer holidays."

I looked at her and said, "Actually, we have only been there once before."

I had spoken to my nurse and physiotherapist about going. They both thought it would be good for me to have a change of scenery; as long as Lotte was there to keep an eye on me. That settled it. I would use this time to prove that I didn't need anyone to look after me. I was capable of looking after myself.

Lotte booked us a room in a small, private guesthouse on the edge of town and we arrived there in time for a late dinner after which we made a small tour of the town before returning to our room for a well-earned rest. Lotte was worn out from the long drive and so was I.

Next morning after breakfast, we made the journey to the large beach for which Skagen is well known and we managed to park the car just in front of the sea. Lotte had the honour of pushing the wheelchair loaded not just with me but also with our bags, towels, lunch and bottles of cold water and a borrowed sun umbrella. She managed the first fifty metres on the hard tarmac but as soon as she hit the hot sand we had problems. The more she pushed the deeper we sank. The sun was burning us and Lotte was soaked with perspiration. Then she decided that the only way we could take our place on the beach was if she carried our belongings separately from the chair to our chosen spot and then returned for me. Once again she tried to push the chair across the sand but it wasn't possible and we started to sink again. The only way would be for me to get out of the chair. Getting up was not difficult but standing up on the sand's unstable surface was. I realised that to maintain my balance I would need to hold on to the chair with my right hand while Lotte held on to the left handle with her left hand. No matter how hard I concentrated and how loud and often I repeated my walking mantra, getting across the sand was a huge challenge. Now I was also sweating like a pig or like somone who had just run a mile in under four minutes!

The physical effort required was triggering repeated spasms in the left side of my body. My brain struggled to try and send messages to my left leg but to no avail. My leg was shaking like an aspen leaf in a summer's breeze. Not only did I have to contend with that but also my left arm was cramping up under my chin. The only way for us to make progress was if Lotte pushed the chair with her left hand and stooping down, held my left leg with her right hand to control the shaking. Luckily for us the sand was more compact and the chair was moving more easily. I was so happy that we had arrived on the beach early and that it wasn't packed with people desperate for sunshine after a particularly long, cold winter.

"Did this spastic leg of yours not come with a user's manual?" Lotte asked from her funny position with her face down by my leg.

"Unfortunately not. It is learning by doing, I guess," I tried to reply while laughing.

I hardly dared think how we looked from a distance, but I did anyway and the picture in my head made me giggle. That set Lotte off as she nearly collapsed onto the sand and she said: "Stop, Charlotte, before it goes too far and you end up wetting yourself." No good, I just started laughing again.

Eventually we made it to a good spot and after spreading ourselves out and getting comfortable we both fell asleep for a couple of hours. When we woke up it was already lunchtime. After lunch, Lotte went for a swim. Our first day on the beach was coming to a close. Probably our passage to the beach taught us both a lesson and to make our leaving easier Lotte decided that she would drive the car over to where we were sitting. Although the beach had filled up there was plenty of space to manoeuvre the car without disturbing anyone. It also saved me the embarrassment of having an audience as I hobbled back across the sand to the car park.

Once back in our room we both showered before taking a quick nap on the beds.

"This trip seems to be turning into a weekend away for old people with all of the naps we are taking," I said, while trying to get dressed.

"We probably both need them but we are still young women and we also need to get dressed up and go out and do some of the things that young women do," Lotte answered with a smile.

Although I was still feeling tired I managed to get dressed. I did not dress in the way I used to, in tight jeans and a T-shirt – because what man would take a second look at a woman in a wheelchair? Lotte pushed me to the restaurant where we had our dinner and then we went on to the harbour for a drink in the cool evening air. We sat down outside a bar and we both gave our orders to the barman. A white wine for Lotte and a fruit juice for me. Lotte left me alone while she went to the bathroom, and I looked around at the busy nightlife.

Suddenly, from out of nowhere, a young man arrived and sat down next to me. I looked over at him from the corner of my eye and saw that he was tall and slim with brown hair. I guessed that he was a couple of years older than me. His presence suddenly made me feel insecure and I crossed my fingers hoping Lotte would soon return. I said to myself, *What does he want? Can't he see that I am sitting in a wheelchair?* Without looking at him I quickly looked around to see to whom I could call for help should I need it. I didn't even know why that thought entered my head.

"Don't we know each other?" he asked me in a quiet voice.

I answered quickly, "I don't think so, I have just had a brain haemorrhage and nearly died so I do not want to listen to you prattle on about nothing."

He stared at me before answering back. "Always up for a fight, now I know that we know each other, Charlotte. I am Frank; we used to play together as children when you visited your grandparents' home in Nibe before they moved. I lived in the long white house opposite them."

Slowly, I turned my head and looked straight at him but avoided eye contact. I did remember a boy named Frank, but I didn't know this young man. I could feel myself starting to blush to my cheeks and I had to pull myself together, before I made eye contact with him.

"Oh sorry, Frank, I do remember you now but maybe it's not the best time for me to bring up my past childhood memories."

He smiled at me. "Don't worry about it, Charlotte. Although I am truly sorry and upset to hear of your brain haemorrhage and that you nearly died, I am so happy to see that you did not and that you have kept your fighting spirit. "Lotte returned and we spent an hour or so talking with Frank. I bought him a beer to apologise and he managed to tell a few stories from my childhood holidays with my grandparents. When the time for him to leave came he gave me a long look before saying to me, "Good luck, Charlotte, and try to remember, next time a young man tries to start a conversation with you not to bite his head off."

I gave him my sweetest crooked smile thinking that there probably wouldn't be a next time.

Later that night, lying in my bed, my body was tired but my brain could not relax. It was full of different thoughts rushing around, such as how lucky I was that Lotte dragged me all the way here kicking and screaming and was taking care of me. I sent a quiet thought to Frank thanking him for not giving up on me and still talking to me even though I was rude to him. I was scared by my own reaction to him earlier that evening, but most of all

I realised that I was more scared about having another haemorrhage and dying. Lying there I also thought of Frank's words about next time and another young man but quickly I pushed those ideas away and convinced myself that there would never be a next time. I would never have a new boyfriend.

"Tough weekend?" Dorte asked me when I turned up for my first physiotherapy session on Monday morning.

"Yes, a bit. I must admit I can still feel the weight of our trip in my body."

She touched my arm. "Tell me about it while I make your stiff muscles relax," she said with a soft and gentle voice that immediately made me feel relaxed. I told her about our expedition to the beach and we both laughed. "Charlotte, walking on sand is twice as difficult and hard for your muscles as walking on a hard surface because you must use more of your strength just to maintain your balance. The cramps you had with your left side were a reaction to the extra effort you put your body through trying to walk on the soft moving surface of the sand."

I responded quickly. "Are you telling me that I am not able to walk on a beach anymore?"

"No, not at all! Just that it will take longer. You keep doing what you are used to and build up strength. But you do need to remember that your body will get tired faster than before."

When our session ended I wheeled myself out onto the terrace to sit in the warm sunshine. I felt the heat put some energy back into my aching limbs. There were two other women sitting at a table close by me drinking coffee and chatting away to each other. I took a guess that they were relatives of another patient and would soon be leaving. As I passed them on my way to my usual corner spot, one of them looked up and asked me, "Are you the teacher we have been told about?" Her remark confused me but made me happy. For the first time since my brain haemorrhage I heard myself being called the teacher and not the woman in the red wheelchair.

Smiling, I looked up at the woman and said, "Yes, that must be me."

She had short brown hair and big brown eyes. "I am sorry. We should introduce ourselves. I am Anita and this is my colleague, Erna. We are teachers at the nearby special needs school but we also handle the daily lessons here in the rehab centre. One of the physiotherapists told us that a young female teacher was staying here for therapy."

I stopped in front of them and we carried on the conversation about teaching and various methods we used to help our students. The conversation not only encouraged me to move my focus from the physical me to the mental me, it also gave me the strength to look at myself as a professional again. They were both warm and nice women, obviously very interested in methods of teaching for people with special needs. Erna ended up by saying, "Come and visit us in the classroom. We can always offer a cup of coffee or tea and maybe continue our discussion about teaching. Or maybe we can convince you to help us?"

As the the short conversation with them had made me feel like a teacher again I was sure we had much more to talk about. I answered without hesitation. "I would love to visit you in the classroom."

20

Charlie Brown

Equilibrium was still my biggest challenge. One morning Dorte started our session saying: "Charlotte, you need to buy some more substantial footwear to give you a solid base and to keep your spastic big toe in the correct position! It will help you to keep your balance."

I looked at her and gave her a big smile. "Sure, Dorte. It is just that substantial footwear is not very sexy." Of course, I knew she was right.

The next day when my parents came to visit we drove to the shopping centre to try to find a pair of training shoes. I wanted to try the big sports shop there. They did have a lot of substantial footwear but as expected nothing was very feminine. The male shop assistant was very nice and found five different pairs for me to try. However, he did not have much empathy with me while I tried them on. It was very difficult for me to get my paralysed foot into the shoe but instead of asking if I needed help, he just grapped my foot and tried to push it into the shoe. It did not hurt at all but it made me feel like a small child unable to dress itself. I felt humiliated and embarrassed that the shop assistant did not get it! Finally, my more practical father got an idea. "Charlotte, let us try to remove the shoelaces and see if the shoe fits the length of your foot." So we did and I picked a new white model with a clear blue logo, 'Nike'. Back at the rehabilitation centre I showed the shoes to Dorte. She did not only approve of the shoes, she also knew a trick of how to put in the shoelaces again so I could manage to close them with one hand. I told her about the humiliating experience in the shop.

She looked at me and responded: "I am sure it was! Charlotte, you have to be prepared for a lot of humiliating experiences in the future. Try not to collect them!"

Later the same day my parents and I were sitting in my room having a coffee when there was a knock on the door and a man entered. He was no one that I recognised and thought that because of his casual way of dressing he must be a relative of another patient. He was wearing white jeans, white trainers and a loose stonewash pale turquoise pullover. I guessed that he must be about forty years of age. He had a round face topped by neatly cut brown hair, but most striking was the pair of intense grey-blue eyes. There was something about his appearance and manner that made me change my mind. He must be a new doctor.

"Hello, Charlotte. My name is Stig and I am the

department's neuropsychologist. My work here is to carry out some tests on your brain to see if you are suffering from any brain damage due to the internal bleeding or resulting from the surgery carried out on you afterwards." I looked up into his eyes and without wanting to I gave him a big smile. He smiled back at me as he continued, "Please will you come to my office at 9.30 am tomorrow? You will find it next to the schoolroom." Just as soon as he arrived he was gone. I found myself giving a long, lingering look at the door he had just disappeared behind and I could sense how empty the room felt without his presence.

I looked over to my mother and said out loud what I was thinking: "That is the man I would like to marry!"

My mother just laughed at me and looked imploringly at my father as she answered: "Okay, darling, let's see if you have any brain damage first and then we can talk about this later."

I remember thinking that my mother really believed that I had suffered from some brain damage. Nevertheless, that man really made a huge impression on me. I guessed that all the way home my mother would talk about her worries. My father would have to reassure her but his words would have no impact on her. As a silent apology to my father I gave him a large smile. Inside I did not care what she thought. I just knew that I wanted to see that man again and could not wait until the next morning.

I was sitting outside his office at 9.30 am sharp. Tentatively I knocked on the door which he opened immediately. Just like yesterday he was casually dressed in white jeans and trainers but today he had on a blue shirt, the colour of which highlighted the blue of his eyes. The shirtsleeves were rolled up just below his elbows and I noticed the soft gold of his skin for the first time. I was also dressed in blue, shorts and T-shirt, and wearing my new trainers. I knew this clothing was easily the most practical for me in the hot weather, but I just did not feel very attractive. I must admit I had thought about wearing something else, maybe a dress, but then realised that in the hospital, my wardrobe choices were very limited, regardless of the fact that I could never attract this man's interest and that those intensive grey-blue eyes would see right through me.

I wheeled myself into position at one end of his large desk when I heard his soft voice, "Charlotte, please move round so that you are on the opposite side of the desk facing me."

My heart said that he did not want me sitting so close to him but common sense told me it was so that he was able to watch my face while we were going through the various procedures. Sitting down opposite me he pushed his chair a little further back and crossed his legs so that his left ankle was resting on his right knee. I noticed immediately that he was wearing a pair of green knitted socks. I looked up away from him and saw the sun shining on the grass of the gardens and thought, *who on earth wears knitted socks on a hot summer's day?* Obviously this man did of course. The man with the grey-blue eyes and the pleasant voice.

Before we began testing Stig asked me a number of questions about my life in general, such as: 'How old are you?'; 'Where do you live?'; 'What is the standard of your education and where do you work?'. During all of this time he never took his eyes off me. Or was it that I never stopped looking into his eyes? I did know that I just loved to hear his voice and I tried to respond to him as quickly and precisely as possible.

Suddenly I could hear myself saying: "I do best in cost-benefit relations." Where did that come from? I did not even know what it meant and I had no idea what his last question was.

Fortunately he just smiled at me. "Sorry, I don't understand. Let us take a short break before the tests and we can return and talk about it again a little later?" We sat in silence for a moment. Maybe it was only for a minute or two but there was no awkwardness to it; just safe, comfortable and relaxing. I took the time to collect my thoughts and looked out of the window. He used the time to prepare the tests.

"Charlotte, in the first test I would like you to memorise the following words: house, dog, autumn and remember them while I ask you questions about this picture."

He had just placed it on the desk in front of me. Easy, I thought. It was not a problem for me to answer his questions about the picture or to remember the three words, but I needed to concentrate hard. My head was full of questions I would have liked to ask this sexy neuropsychologist sitting in front of me, questions such as: How old are you?; Are you married? Questions I knew that I could never ask and I was convinced that even if I did he would never answer them anyway.

The second test was for dexterity. He gave me some red and white bricks and a picture with two different patterns.

"Please look at the pattern and then construct it using the bricks."

It was hard for me and and made my hand sweat. He knew it was difficult for me and again we took another break before the third test. Again we sat in silence. I could not help thinking that maybe the breaks were some kind of test, too? For the third test he showed me a picture of a man.

"Charlotte, look at this man and try to remember his face. Later on you will have to point him out in a bigger picture."

Easy, I thought, and hardly looked at the picture of the man. Then he placed the bigger picture in front of me.

"Please point out the man."

Now I was breaking out in a sweat trying hard to concentrate. I took a long time just staring at the various people in the large picture but I could not recognise the one that I was looking for. Eventually, I gave up. I was so upset by my failure at such a relatively simple task. Stig smiled at me.

"Do not worry. We'll take a break and try again in a few minutes."

Test number four was the same as number three but

this time it was the face of a woman. It took me a while but eventually I found the correct match and gave a big sigh of relief as he said: "We are finished." Stig looked through his papers for a few minutes before he spoke.

"You are suffering from a mild form of 'Prosopagnose' which means that you have difficulty in recognising people's faces. Apart from that your neurological function is fine."

I was not listening very attentively. I just wanted to turn my chair and escape from this man and room. Just as I reached for the door handle he asked me another question, one which made me stop and take notice.

"When are you planning to return to work again?"

Before I could answer this I turned my chair to face him again. I used the time to formulate my reply. "I begin in August when the children return to school from their summer holidays."

He nodded. "Good, and what kind of Charlotte can they expect to find?"

I thought it was such a stupid thing to ask but as I thought it through, I came to the conclusion that he was one of the few people prepared to talk to me about leaving, and returning to work and life outside again.

"They can expect Charlotte, just with a paralysed arm."

I could not prevent the smile that came to my lips as I turned again to leave him. Leaving the office I made my way out to my favourite corner of the terrace. Here I tried to get a hold of myself and put my emotions into some perspective. I was wondering what went on in his office? Why couldn't I concentrate on the questions he was asking me? All I could think about was how it would feel to be kissed by a man at least ten years older than me. I suddenly felt insecure and nervous, all of these strange thoughts running through my head. Perhaps I did have some brain damage? Maybe they did not want to tell me! I sat outside watching the ripples playing across the surface of the lake. It took more than an hour before I felt calm enough and able to think rationally again. I looked around just to make certain that I was alone and that no one would be able to hear me before saying to myself: "No, Charlotte, you do not have brain damage, you have just fallen for this man whom you know nothing about!"

21

On a mission

For the next couple of days I was a woman on a mission, seeking to find out all I could about this man, who, like nobody before, had filled my head with such a passion and I must admit not only my head but my heart also. The first person I got the chance to interrogate was, of course, Dorte. As she was working on stretching the muscles in my left leg I asked: "That neuropsychologist who interviewed me the other day, do you know him?"

She looked up at me and replied: "Sorry, Charlotte, I am still fairly new here and have not yet come into contact with him. I am sure that Lasse knows him because he has worked here for years."

"It's not important," I quickly responded.

I did not want her to mention it to anyone. Another way of getting the information had just come to mind.

The next morning I took the opportunity to visit Anita and Erna in the schoolroom. I was hoping that they would have some information on the neuropsychologist who worked next door. There was only one student present that day so they had plenty of time to talk to me. I spent some time looking at the various materials that they used for teaching and we spoke of the different style of teaching in this type of environment when suddenly, Erna said: "Charlotte, as you are younger than both Anita and me maybe you will be more help to Kirsten here with her book report." With these words I let myself be pursuaded to help the patient. Kirsten was a fifteen-year-old girl with a broken back from a car accident. Sitting there in the wheelchair teaching this young student made me think. I somehow had a leg on both sides: I had my education and a few years of experience as a teacher, and my new experience of being disabled. Even though I was enjoying the opportunity to relate to my profession again, I had another motive for my visit and had to try to find the right moment to bring it up.

It came shortly afterwards. I was laughing quite loudly at something Anita had just told me. I stopped myself.

"Maybe we should be quiet if the neuropsychologist is working with a patient next door?"

Anita answered immediately. "Don't worry, Stig is not in today."

I looked first at Anita then at Erna. "Okay then, I do not need to worry!"

Erna looked at Anita and asked, "Has he gone to Spain?" Anita shook her head for a no and explained: "Stig's hobby is to find, buy and import wine from Spain. Which he then sells in his spare time." I smiled and tried my best not to look too interested. "He is not in Spain. He is just out for a meeting in town today."

I guessed that as they referred to him by name and knew all about his wine importing, they had to know him fairly well. After my somewhat clumsy attempt to keep the conversation about him, I only discovered that they had had the occasional coffee together. Putting two and two together, Anita then asked, "Why do you want to know about Stig?"

I blushed because I had been caught out and gave a funny answer. "I have a thing about psychologists and would like to try to devise some test to try out on him."

Anita looked at me and gave me a wink. I made my goodbyes and left.

A few days passed and I was invited to try some silk screen-printing in the occupational therapy room. Everyone participating in this work had been in the centre longer than I had and they all knew Stig. With great difficulty, I managed to control my tongue and carried on trying to master the art of silk screen-printing. I was not sure if it was that I had only the use of one hand, I was missing any creativity or that it was just plain difficult but my colourful parrot turned into a shot canary peeing itself. I received no admiring comments from my fellow artists. It did not matter to me. I knew exactly what I was going to do with it.

Next morning I wheeled myself to the first floor and up to the classroom door. I listened at the keyhole to make certain they were occupied. Then I moved over to the next office and tapped gently on the door. I was hoping that he was not occupied with another patient. Luck was on my side for once and soon a smiling Stig opened the door. I was so nervous that my palms were sweating as I handed him the silk print. "It is my turn to test you. What is this?" Before he even had the chance to answer I wheeled myself down the corridor towards the lift. I could feel his eyes on me but he did not say anything. I did not turn round to look at him. Back outside in my little corner of the terrace where the warm sun shined on me and the ripples on the lake tried to calm me, I felt nothing but negative thoughts. How could I be so stupid? To him I was just another patient. There was no reason for him to notice me. Why should he? He could not even see my best feature, a small, neat bum, because I spent all of my time sitting in my Ferrari red wheelchair.

The day after, on my return from physiotherapy, I saw an envelope leaning against a bottle of body lotion on my bedside cabinet. I pushed myself over and ripped it open. I pulled out a folded sheet of paper. My heart was beating so fast and I could hear the blood thundering in my ears as it rushed through my body.

Dear Charlotte

I do not know who is testing whom but I do know that I like receiving presents from the young red-haired woman in the Ferrari red chair who makes me feel like Charlie Brown.

Stig

"What?" I said as the breath I had not realised I was holding shot from my mouth. My little test made him take notice of me. He liked me! At least in the way Charlie Brown likes the little red-haired girl who was always biting the end of her pencil in the cartoon series. These few lines had the power to make me believe. I was now a woman with a future. I folded the note and put it into my pocket. I sent a silent 'thank you' to Frank from Skagen. Maybe there would be a next time, after all?

It was now my fourth week at the rehabilitation centre and on Monday morning my sister arrived. Vibsen was spending a week staying with our parents before her husband and their children would come to spend the holidays with her in-laws. I was happy to see her again and it was very nice for me to experience both her and my brother's commitment and support towards me during this difficult phase in my life. Later that same Monday the head of the department walked into my room.

"Good to find you here, Charlotte, I have some good news for you. The department is due to close for the summer holidays from this Friday and we aim to discharge as many patients as possible. Based on the information I have from both your physiotherapist and neuropsychologist we have decided to discharge you into your parents' care. We have arranged for you to visit the rehab unit twice a week in Aalborg to continue your exercise programme."

I barely heard what she was telling me because I could only think what the neuropsychologist had been saying about me. I wanted to tell her that I needed to have another test. Was that true or was it just because I wanted to see him again? I had to take control of this situation now I was back on my own. I would have to make a plan to get to see him again.

22

Back as an adult

It was the last day at the rehabilitation centre, four months after my brain haemorrhage and the first day of my new life. It was time to say goodbye to this wonderful place. I could hardly believe that out little country had a place like this. Vibsen came to collect my few belongings and me. Before leaving I had one last session with Dorte.

"Charlotte, take care of yourself and fight for being who you are and for what you want!" Dorte told me as her farewell. I felt very emotional when I gave her a last hug goodbye.

"Dorte, you have been such a great help to me both physically and mentally."

Vibsen and I left for the drive to my brother's workplace. She parked the car just outside the main entrance and took out first the wheelchair then me.

She helped me from the car using the armrest of the wheelchair for support. We made our way to the reception desk and asked the woman there to tell Peter that his sisters had arrived. I took a deep breath as Vibsen gently lifted my hand from the safety of the chair and pulled it away from me. I wobbled a little as I needed to get my balance before I could take my first faltering step down the long corridor. Peter was now standing waiting for me outside his office. My movements were neither elegant nor beautiful but with each slow, stiff step I moved forward towards him. Peter was standing with arms outstretched waiting to hug me when I reached him, or to catch me should I fall. I was not going to fall. I concentrated so hard that it made my head spin. I worked so much that I could feel the rivers of perspiration running down my back. From the corner of my eye I saw Vibsen pushing the wheelchair in time with my steps. Just as I reached Peter my legs were shaking under me. Vibsen saw it and placed the wheelchair right behind me. As soon as I felt the chair behind my knees I sank back into it, maybe not gracefully, but more of a flop back into it. Nevertheless, I had made my first walk in public without a mishap. Peter, Vibsen and the receptionist gave me a round of applause and I blushed with embarrassment. I called my thanks to the woman at the front desk and wheeled myself into the office. We had arrived in time for lunch. Peter had the boardroom table prepared for us with some of my favourites, such as hard-boiled eggs with mayonnaise. I enjoyed my lunch of rye bread and eggs, fresh sun-ripe tomatoes and crispy cucumbers. For me it was the perfect reward for my hard work.

We sat eating and talking for over an hour discussing my future plans.

"I hope to go back to work in August. I will look for a place to live nearby the school so I will have no problems about transport."

I was pleased that they listened to my plan without interruption and felt that at last I was back on an even footing with my siblings. We were all equal again.

After our lunch Vibsen and I made the drive back to our parents' house in Løgstør. Here, as at Peter's office, she parked the car near the front gate and helped me out. She held my arm for me until I was comfortable with my balance. This time she did not take the wheelchair. I looked over at the front door and suddenly it seemed so much smaller than I remembered. Why was the postbox set in the middle, in front of the three steps leading up to the door, making access even more restricted? Again, I was concentrating hard to climb the steps and, of course, my paralysed arm decided that now was the perfect time to make its presence felt. Only this time it did not cramp up under my cheek because I hit the bottom of the bloody postbox. I could feel my sister's hand on the small of my back and was not sure if it was to support me or push me forward. I felt like I should be saying 'ouch' but was my brain working properly? I noticed that I was not feeling any pain even when I saw small drops of blood beading on my skin. I felt nothing. My sister, standing behind me, immediately removed her hand from my back.

"Don't worry, I can't feel anything. My arm will not pass because it is caught on the side of the mailbox. Please, just help me by pressing my arm down." Very carefully she put her hand on my paralysed arm but it did not move at all. I turned my head to look at her and wheezed at her: "Put some muscle in it. Push harder!" I felt her push a bit harder.

"Are you sure it is not hurting?" she asked.

"No, just push!"

Finally, she took a firmer hold on my arm and pushed down with all her strength. At last my arm moved and I could pass by and get into the house. Unfortunately my parents had heard the commotion. My dad opened the kitchen door as I limped through the house.

"Hi, Dad. Today is 31 July 1989. You owe me an all-expenses-paid holiday in France!"

He gave me a hug. "Yes and you so deserve it!"

I felt the sweat all over my body and how tired I was in my legs. It might not be a 'Dream Mile' but it was good enough to get me to France.

It was my first weekend out of the rehabilitation centre and I was spending it with Peter and his wife, Marie, at their house in Skive. Marie picked me up at my parents' house on Friday evening. When we arrived at Peter's I was still angry with him because we had not been able to talk about his interference in my financial affairs. So, as soon I saw him I asked, "Why did you talk to my bank?"

He looked as though he was expecting my question and answered immediately.

"I went to the bank to make certain that your former landlord had repaid your deposit. I thought that you would prefer me rather than Mum and Dad to do it?"

I looked down. "Of course I did. I am sorry for overreacting."

That Friday evening we spent our time talking about my future. I asked them, "Can you take me to Åbybro tomorrow morning? I have heard from a colleague that there is a small house for rent just across from the school and I have been in contact with the agent about taking on a lease. The housing association has phoned to say that I could view the house this Saturday morning."

They both nodded and said: "Of course we will."

Early next morning the three of us set off to meet the agent and viewed what I hoped would become my new home.

The house was situated on the old road between Åbybro and Aalborg almost opposite the school. The house was compact and neat. It consisted of a living room with an open-plan kitchen, one bedroom and bathroom and a small garden. Perfect for me and I agreed to rent the house immediately. Peter's only concern was for the garden.

"Charlotte, you are not the most green-fingered person I know."

I laughed. He was so right.

"I will ask the handyman at the school to help me."

He smiled before adding, "Our next and biggest challenge will be to convince our anxious mother that you are ready to start your life again and be an independent woman once more."

We drove over to visit our parents and Peter was right. My decision as predicted made our mother worried about me living alone. She had to give in when our father gave his blessing to the idea and Marie gave the perfect argument. "Charlotte has to try to live on her own to see what she can handle!"

On Monday morning Marie drove me to the town hall in Åbybro. I needed to meet with my social worker, who explained to me the help that I was entitled to now. Whether I liked it or not I was a full blown 'social case'. Our next port of call was the housing association where in exchange for a hefty deposit I received the keys to my new home. It was a strange feeling; here I was about to start again as an independent woman and I had to rely on my family to do a lot of the necessary work that moving entailed.

23

Back at school

Finally, I got the opportunity to visit the school and meet with my colleagues. Everyone was busy with preparations for the new school year but they all took the time to welcome me back. It felt a bit awkward to be back at the school. It did help a lot to talk to my boss about my new duties and what he expected from me.

"Charlotte, I am very happy to see you return to work as we planned. But I have to be realistic about your strengths and weaknesses, and make certain that you are not overstretched too soon. I have decided and already spoken to your colleague you used to share the class with. We have worked out a plan. Although she is really a part-time teacher, she has agreed to work extra hours to be a 'shadow' for you. If the work becomes too much and you get tired she will take over and you can return home to rest. This is how we shall work until you are able to resume working full time again."

I was very happy about the plan and I gave him a big smile and a 'Thank you!'

The following weekend I was due to move in and the family came to help transfer my belongings from the school storeroom and into my new home. Of course, I was unable to do much and so I spent some time walking from home to the school so that I could have an idea of just how much time I would need to get to work. It also gave me the opportunity to reread the note that I had received from Stig. Back from my second crossing of the road I had to acknowledge the fact that I was tired. I dropped like a stone onto my new white two-seater sofa to rest. Just as I closed my eyes there was a knock at the door.

"Hello, may we enter?"

It was my friend Tine and her husband, Jens. They had rented a house just outside Åbybro. Jens was starting work at the boarding school in town. I was so happy to know that they would be close by to me. Tine busied herself making coffee, tea and slicing a home-baked cake that she had brought with her. Everyone took the opportunity to take a well-earned break. As we all sat around the table, Tine raised her cup towards mine and offered the toast. "Welcome back. It is good to have you home again."

I smiled at her thinking just how right she was. Charlotte was back. That evening when everything in the house was in order, the bed was made and even the fridge was full of my favourite orange yogurt we made the drive back to our parents' house. We had a late dinner and I spent the night in their home.

The next morning the phone rang and Mum rushed to answer the call. I knew that they were talking about me because I heard her responding.

"Yes, she is!"

This was followed by a long silence before I heard her saying to the caller, "If you are not serious about her then just stay away from her."

I was not sure who had called. It could not be Stig because he did not know where I was. That could only mean that maybe the caller was Jesper. From deep within me the outrage that I felt overwhelmed me and without thinking I lashed out and hit her on the arm. It must have hurt her a lot as she dropped the phone and looked very frightenedly at me. At this moment I did not care if I had hurt her. I just screamed.

"How dare you! Who called me?"

"It was Jesper," she quickly answered.

In that split second I decided that now was the time for me to leave as soon as possible and start to rebuild my life without interference from other people. I was so furious. I called for my father and demanded he drove me back to my own house immediately. My mother could not understand that what she had done was wrong nor why I would not stay with them until school started again. She tried.

"What if something happens to you and you need someone in a hurry?"

I answered without looking at her, "Then I will call Tine!"

As a compromise and to make them drive me home I accepted food from them. With Mum's home-made meatballs (always a favourite of mine) and a pile of freshly laundered clothes in hand we made the journey. It was late Sunday evening when I finally unlocked the door of my new home. Eventually my parents left and for the first time in so long I was alone in a quiet house. I started to get a little worried but forced myself to sit for an hour in the living room without putting on the light. I needed to get used to being on my own again and reminded myself that Tine was close if I needed anything. What could happen to me now that the worst had already happened? Life must go on. I was going forward and not backwards from now on. Exhausted, I finally forced myself into bed and crawled under the duvet just in time as my eyes closed and I fell into a deep sleep.

Monday morning arrived and I woke fully rested after ten hours of heavy sleep. Not only did I wake fully refreshed but I was full of energy and ready to take on life and whatever it threw at me. I ate breakfast still wearing pyjamas sitting on my white sofa and looked intently round the room. The sofa was placed against the wall between my bedroom and sitting room. It was from this spot that I could see most of my little house. To my left was the door out into the garden and through it I could see the school and the surrounding green fields. Through this door the morning sun flowed in quickly warming the room. Across the room and just in front of my kitchen was the round white dining table and its four matching chairs. When I turned my head to the right I could see the small entrance hall and front door. The house was full of light and warmth and was my little piece of paradise. I loved it. Now all I needed to do was find a way of getting in touch with Stig again, but how, I had no idea. Finally, I got up and made my way to the bathroom to shower and get dressed. I was not only surprised but also shocked when I discovered just how long this simple act took me. I would need to be out of bed before sunrise to be at work for 8 am.

Just as I was about to flop back down on the sofa there was a knock on the door. Tine called out as she pushed it open.

"Hi, Charlotte, I just have time for a quick cup of tea before I need to go and collect Jens from school. Today we have an appointment with the bank to see about a mortgage, as we want to start looking for our own house to buy."

Although I was always very happy to see Tine this visit was unexpected and I had to ask the question. "Did my mother send you?"

Laughing, Tine turned to go into the kitchen to make the tea.

"This should be your job, Charlotte, as you're the host. You should be making the tea!"

I smiled towards the kitchen. "Yes, but if you only have time for a quick cup..." I left the sentence unfinished and we carried on with our usual ping-pong conversation. While we sat drinking our tea I told her how long it had taken for me to shower and dress in the morning and just how frustrated it made me feel. It helped a lot for me to just say these words and get it off my chest. Tine had no answer, but at least now I had voiced my frustrations I could relax a little. I also took the opportunity to tell her about the neuropsychological tests I went through, and about Stig and his letter. Finally, I told her how desperate I was to contact him again but did not know how to go about it. Tine gave me a look.

"Listen to yourself. If I didn't know you better I would think you were full of self-pity. What would you have done before your haemorrhage?"

With these words echoing in my ears she stood up and made herself ready to leave. In my haste to show her out I got up too quickly and almost fell on top of her. She gave me a grin, slapped my backside with the flat of her hand and walked to the door.

"Charlotte, you need to continue with your exercises every day. Maybe just walking up and down the garden path will help strengthen your muscles and maintain your balance!"

She closed the door behind her and I fell back onto the sofa again. I knew that she was right and that she had helped me put things into perspective. I needed to get my act together and not fall into the trap of self-pity. It was me and me only who could get my life on track. Basically, I did not believe that life gave anyone a challenge bigger than they could handle. This was my challenge and I would deal with it.

The first few days in my new home I spent a lot of time practising getting in and out of bed and getting myself dressed ready for work within an hour. Every day I walked across the road to the school where my colleagues were busying themselves as the school reopened the following week. I was certain that I was in the way as I dragged myself around. But they all tried to include me in the preparations. I was having problems relating to my work and kept on finding other things to do. Should I write to Stig? Maybe he would be able to put me back on the right track. At least I could use this as an excuse. I wrote him a postcard to his workplace and included my new address. Now the ball was back in his court.

Day by day, I gradually took on more responsibility for planning my own classes and I was shattered by the time I made my way to bed at night. I was not eating properly and most of my meals seemed to consist of yogurt. I was so pleased to be back at work again that I did not worry about food.

24

The taxi driver

As well as starting back to work I was beginning my new physiotherapy regime with help from the staff at Aalborg. I was taken there by a local taxi. The nice taxi driver said on my first trip, "Charlotte, if you need a car as a private taxi, you just call me on this private telephone line. I will give you a fair price." His words gave me an idea.

So, the day before the school reopened I booked him to drive me to the bus station in Aalborg. As we approached the bridge on the Aalborg-Nørresundby road he turned off the meter even though we still had some more kilometres to travel. I looked at him.

"Thank you very much!"

He looked back with a large smile. "It's nothing. I am happy to be able to help someone trying to start a new life and overcoming health problems on the way."

I arrived in time to catch the bus to Viborg. On my

arrival there I bumped into two elderly women. One of them called my name. I looked up and I saw they were my aunts, my father's two sisters. Damn! They were sure to tell my parents that they had seen me in Viborg and I was not ready to tell my parents about Stig. I could see the look of curiosity in their eyes and quickly thought of an excuse for my being there.

"Oh, hello, Aunt Eva and Aunt Lise. I am on my way to the hospital for some physiotherapy. What are you both doing in Viborg?"

Aunt Eva answered. "We are waiting for the bus to Vejle. We are staying with your Aunt Marie for a few days."

I gave them my best weapon, a large smile.

"Okay, give her my love and try not to drink too much."

They giggled and I could see their bus approaching the stop. I waited until they were on board before sighing with relief. At least I had got away with my ruse. Making my way to the taxi rank I turned a little fast and had to struggle to keep my balance but I managed. I waved at a taxi. It was only when I was sitting in the back of the taxi I realised just how hot and sweaty I was. I could also feel my arm begin to cramp and lift itself up to my chin as it did when I sneezed, got nervous or put too much pressure on my body. With all of the strength in my right arm I managed to lower it down just as we arrived in front of the rehabilitation department. As I left the taxi I glanced at the dashboard clock and saw that it was twelve o' clock; lunchtime. Without planning, I had arrived at the best time as there would be no one around to see me. I felt like a thief as I sneaked into the building and made my way straight to the lift. I tried to be as silent as possible but my arm was cramping again and my left leg was dragging behind me across the hard surface of the floor.

Luckily, without meeting anyone, I arrived at Stig's office and knocked on his door. Quickly he opened it, almost as though he was expecting me. He did not look at all surprised to find me at his door. He just ushered me in closing the door behind me.

"Sorry, but this is not a good time for me, Charlotte. I have to be in a meeting in half an hour."

Then he told me to sit down in one of the two couches placed at the other end of his long office. I swore that I never saw them during my last visit. We had only just sat down when there was a tap on the door. Stig got up to go and open it. A tall, good-looking young boy walked in. I guessed he was about fifteen years of age. I was not very surprised when he said, "Stigsen, I have to collect the key." It was when he finished the sentence with, "… for mother" that I felt as if a bucket of cold water had been thrown over me. In a hurry Stig found and handed the key to the boy, who left just as quietly as he had come in.

"Was that your son?" I blurted out.

"Yes, the youngest. I have another son . He is seventeen years old." He answered me without looking at me. Suddenly the situation changed. It was like we were two strangers who had just met, exchanging information about our respective families. Stig sat down next to me and looked at his watch. Then he stood again and said: "I have to go to the meeting. I will drive you."

In silence we made our way to his car which was parked in front of the building. Quickly he cleared the front passenger seat so that I could sit down. All the while he was looking over his shoulder or at his watch. He seemed stressed and anxious. I wanted to try to relax him and said, "Just drop me off in town. I want to do some shopping."

He drove us through some streets that I had never been through. He stopped the car in the square where the sign said 'Nytorv'. As I left the car I turned to him and asked, "Are you married?"

He did not look at me. "Yes, for now," was the reply. He spoke the words almost in a whisper. I just stood there looking at him for what seemed a long time before I turned and walked away from the car. I did not look back when I heard the car pull away from the kerb. Part of me was disappointed but the other part was happy that he did not cancel his meeting just because I had unexpectedly turned up. I went directly to the bus station and found a bus back to Aalborg.

25

A home visit

The following Monday on my return from work I found the letter waiting for me in my mailbox. It was a short note from Stig. All it said was that he had been haunted by the look I gave him as we parted in Nytorv. If I did not object he would come and visit me on Thursday before lunch. At work I told them a small lie that I had a home visit from the hospital and as the appointment time was not definite I would need to take the whole day off on Thursday. It was not a complete lie. I was going to have a visit at home and he was working at a hospital.

Finally, the day arrived at last. I had slept until 9 am, as ever it took me a while to shower and dress, so I did not have too much time to sit and think before Stig arrived at 11.20 am. As he walked up the path to my front door I could see that intense look in his eyes. I was watching him through the round glass window and I noticed he was carrying a large box in his arms. Flustered I unlocked and opened the door just as he was about to struggle to ring the bell.

"Come in to my little paradise." He put the box down on the table. "Are you moving in?" I asked surprised.

"Not yet," came the reply. He looked at me. "I wasn't sure if you had enough food in the house and so I have brought us lunch."

From the box he brought out bread, butter, ham and two bottles of Spanish Cava. I was confused by this and reminded him, "I am not allowed to drink alcohol for a year."

He smiled. "Okay, then we can save it until you can drink it."

Was that his way of telling me that he wanted to be with me? I gave him a smile and leaned against the table as he put the box down onto the floor. He stood up and put his arms around me and gave me the softest and most intense kiss I have ever had. It felt so right.

Later, while we were sitting on the sofa eating our lunch, I asked him, "Where are you supposed to be today?"

"I told them at work that I had a brain injury conference in Århus to attend. I hate to lie but with my marriage in such a mess I had to escape and see you. Charlotte, this is my choice and I will have to live with the consequences. My old boss always said it can lead to a life of endless unhappiness not to choose well, whilst a good choice can end the unhappiness."

As Stig leaned closer to me, I could just hear him mumbling, "Clever man, the old boss," as his soft lips brushed against mine.

For the next four hours we had together we never moved from the sofa. I had never before met a man who could look at me and look through me at the same time. Never before had I met someone who I could have such inspiring conversations with for hours on end. I may have laughed before but I have never felt happier and more alive than I felt that afternoon. When the time came for him to leave he said, "Your world is so simple and easy."

Through the window I watched him get into his car and drive away. Even after our conversation and kisses I did not know if I would ever see him again. The waiting was excruciating but it was sweetened almost every day with the arrival of a short note from him. Besides a lot of sweet talk they also contained Stig's feelings of remorse especially towards his two sons.

Despite my long-held decision that I would never be unfaithful, l I found myself as the 'other woman' in Stig's infidelity. There was nothing I could do but wait for him. I was only really happy when we were together. This was a position in my life that I was not happy with. If it was true that his marriage was over I had decided that I would fight for him and for our blossoming love. One evening, a few days after Stig's visit, Lotte phoned me and she soon realised that I was not sounding my usual carefree self. Slowly she coaxed me to tell her what was happening with my life and the role that Stig was playing. She shocked me by the vehemence of her response. "Get rid of him. A married man is the last person you need in your life."

26

All alone

Friday came round again and some of my colleagues asked me about my plans for the weekend. Although it was normal for us to discuss them, this time it seemed to me that I was the only person being asked the question. Even Tine phoned to invite me to stay with her and her husband. She tried to persuade me by saying, "You will not only have company, you will get home-cooked food."

I had to lie to her. "Tine, it is tempting but I am going to visit Peter and Marie this weekend."

Instead, when I returned home that afternoon, I locked the front door and unplugged the phone. I had decided to spend the weekend on my own. This turned out to be the longest weekend of my entire twenty-five years. I told myself several times, *if you cannot be alone with yourself, you cannot expect others to be with you*.

The only time I moved from my sofa was when I got up for more yogurt, used the bathroom or went to bed. My small twenty-two-inch television was playing all of the time and I worried that it might burn itself out. Around midnight on Saturday I felt restless and unable to relax. I was having long conversations trying to convince myself that it was not a good idea for me to be in a relationship with a married man. *Charlotte, do not be stupid. No matter what he tells you, he will never leave his wife and children for you!* By 3 am I was desperate. I got up and went to the bathroom. I stared at myself in the wall mirror and had the same conversation over again. I knew that I could call Tine whatever the time was. She would hurry over to me. This knowledge helped me get back some perspective in my life. I did not phone her but went back to bed. On Sunday I spent most of my time sleeping. By the time Monday morning arrived, I had slept for at least eighteen hours. I was the first to arrive at the school and felt full of energy and desperate for some conversation with another human. Finally, I was in the classroom with the children and as usual I started the week by asking each one of them to tell us what they had done over the weekend. This Monday morning I let them talk for a much longer time than usual. I enjoyed it so much listening to other voices than my own.

It was fantastic being back at work and I started off each morning happy and full of energy. Quickly, though, I began to tire. Then I felt worried about concentrating on my teaching, particularly when I started to think about Stig but also because my brain was tired. Luckily for me my colleagues understood and they did not expect anything extra from me. My shadow just appeared and took over from me. Between us we did not let the children or the school down. Try as I might, I could not rediscover the teacher I used to be. The children had also noticed the changes. One morning a girl who was usually the quietest of them all suddenly raised her hand.

"Why are you always sitting down? You never move around as you used to. Your voice is so boring now."

Those words coming from her were unexpected, and they hurt. I tried to smile as I remembered the old saying 'From the mouths of babes and innocents'. I clearly remembered my own definition of a good teacher: it was someone who was 'physically active and with an outgoing personality who had the ability to inspire their pupils'. I was unable to do this now. I needed to be seated at my desk or if not, at least perched on the edge of it to keep my balance. My voice was somnolent and boring. I knew no medicine in the world could bring back the teacher I used to be.

27

Because I can

The following weekend I again started using white lies to be on my own. Firstly Tine called and invited me over. I told her that I was visiting my parents. Then my mother phoned and asked if I wanted them to come over and pick me up so that I could spend some time with them? I told her that I would be spending the weekend with Tine. I was surprised that I felt the need to lie to people who loved me. Especially my mother who still could not see me as an independent woman but only as her twenty-five-year-old baby daughter.

As soon as I got home on Friday lunchtime, I telephoned my friendly taxi driver and told him my plans. He liked to be able to help me on my adventures. This time I needed him to take me to the train station in Aalborg and to pick me up from the station after midnight. He collected me from home and we drove to the station in Aalborg, where I got the 1 pm train to København. Five hours later I arrived at my destination. On arrival I got off the train to visit the bathroom. In the bathroom I looked in the mirror and said out loud, "I took the train to København on my own. Just because I can!" Then I went to the shop to buy water and fruit for my trip back.

I had noticed something when I caught the train from Aalborg. The left side of my body was not feeling as brave as the rest of me. I had felt my left side become frozen with fear and as always my left arm cramped up under my chin. It made it difficult for me to climb the narrow, high steps up into the train. Also, vibrations from the train made it difficult for me to maintain my balance and stand. So I needed to be seated for the whole journey. Fortunately for me I could smile. It was a little crooked but still it was recognised as a smile and not a grimace. In spite of my travel companions' general Friday fatigue they were quite happy to sit and chat with me. On the way back we had just left Odense where most of the passengers I had talked to got off and were replaced by a new group. Suddenly, I felt a strong pain in my head just behind my right ear. It used all of my energy just to force myself to breathe. Sweat was beginning to trickle down my back and I felt my palms begin to get moist. I could even feel beads of perspiration form on my upper lip. I looked around at the other passengers to see if they had noticed any change in me. They all seem preoccupied with various activities. I could see a man on the other side of the train watching me and smiling at me. Maybe it was only because I was staring at him? I realised that I was on my own. That made me scared. What if my blood pressure was getting too high? What if I lost the ability to speak? To make sure I had not I whispered to myself, "My name is Charlotte." There was no reaction from the people sitting around me. I continued saying it in English, then German and lastly French. I convinced myself that if I could continue repeating the sentence in various languages I was not having another brain haemorrhage. Eventually, the train arrived at Kolding. I must have seemed like a nun chanting as the person next to me gave me a peculiar look. I gave him a shy smile. I knew in the future I would be frightened every time I felt a headache coming on. I comforted myself with the fact that if I could repeat a sentence in a variety of languages then I would be okay. Furthermore, I'd like to think people around me would help me just as Jesper did if anything happened to me. We arrived in Århus and the man sitting next to me, much to his relief I suspected, got off. The seat was taken by an elderly woman. She talked to me all the way to Aalborg occupying my mind and relieving me of my anxious thoughts.

By the time we had arrived in Aalborg and I was sitting in the taxi I was almost crying. I was so tired. My nice driver looked at me.

"Did you have a nice trip?"

I looked back at him with a feeling of relief and a wonderful sense of pride in my achievement. "I did. I am just so tired I could cry."

He gave me a large smile. "You cry if you need to. I will take you back home. Did you meet anyone in København?"

I managed to keep back the tears. "No, I just went there and back."

He turned his head and looked at me. "Why?"

I gave him a tired and surely wry smile, "Because I can!"

From that moment I decided that my Ferarri red wheelchair would go into retirement.

28

The truth hurts

I was feeling very frustrated by the reactions of one particular child in my class. I was trying so hard to bring back the old Charlotte as a teacher for them. I was working on an alternative teaching method. We had constructed a circus and used clowns and trapeze artists as the important vowels. We had also baked biscuits in the shape of alphabet letters and then eaten them during our break time. Right now I was reading a story aloud to them when that child called out to me, "Your voice is so boring!"

He was right, of course. My voice had changed and instead of rising and falling in tone it was flat and monotonous. I was unable to express emotions with it. His words annoyed and hurt me. Instead of controlling my feelings, for the first time in my teaching career I screamed, "Shut up!"

Shocked by my sudden outburst the whole class fell silent. I looked at the children in front of me. I was confused by what had just happened. They all looked at me with scared faces. I was riddled with guilt for losing control of myself in front of them. It felt like a lump had grown in my throat, and tears were burning in my eyes. Just before I managed to leave the room I whispered, "I am sorry!"

I hid in the bathroom until I was able to control my emotions and was certain I was not going to cry. I had just realised that very moment the unpleasant truth. My body now functioned in a very different way from before. I had to face it. The children were right even though it hurt me. After making sure that I was again in control of my emotions I returned to the classroom and found the children still sitting in stunned silence.

I dragged my chair into the open space in front of the class. I sat down and slowly I spoke.

"As you can see, as a result of a very sudden illness my body has changed. You can see for yourselves that my left arm is paralysed and hangs loosely down my side. If I overwork my body, if I suddenly sneeze or for some reason I become frightened, the muscles will suddenly cramp and tighten pulling my arm up towards my chin. You also see that I am walking slowly and with a limp in my left leg. It is because my left leg is partially paralysed as well."

I paused to give them time to take in my words and to see if they had any questions for me. Nobody moved or said a word. So I continuted slowly.

"You notice that when I am getting tired my smile becomes crooked and some of you have commented that my voice has changed becoming flat and toneless. All of these changes mean that I have to work particularly hard. I use up a lot of energy. It is difficult for me to be the teacher I once was and I am very sad because of it. Sometimes it can make me very angry. I would like you all to try to understand that beneath my changed body I am still the same Charlotte."

They had listened without interruption. I could feel my inner pain slowly change to an inner calm; probably because the situation had become so emotionally charged. I ended up inviting the whole class to stay at my house for a sleepover. The first child to shout out, of course, had to be the one who had said I had a boring voice.

"Please, miss, please, miss, when can we come?"

Just as quickly I answered him without thinking. "If your parents all agree you can come on Friday 2 September."

Before I left work I went to see my boss. I wanted to inform him of the situation in the class; how, in the end, I had invited the children to a sleepover in my house. As always he listened but ended up saying, "Charlotte, remember, it is okay to cancel the sleepover, if it is too much for you to handle."

I stood up to leave and replied without looking at him, "I know but I am not going to cancel."

I was relieved that my honesty seemed to clear the air with the children. Anyhow, I was both nervous and excited at the prospect of them staying over night. I supposed they would all tell their parents what had happened in class. I prepared myself for the negative reactions that were bound to follow. To my joy there were none. In contrast the parents praised me for my honesty and forthright attitude with their children. I felt so relieved that I was working in an environment where my teaching skills were not questioned or doubted, at least not to my face. What they might say behind my back was another matter. I heard nothing on the school's grapevine. My talk with the children had left me with a feeling of relief; even the knowledge that I was more aware of my body and its reactions to outside stimulus. Often when I returned home I felt very tired. Several times I even felt the strong spasms in my leg because I had over exerted it. My nerves kicked in with the thought of the children coming to stay. However, the fact that almost every day I had in my hand a new letter from Stig helped to wash away any feelings of doubt and tiredness.

Do not ask me why, but one day I knew that this was going to be a very important letter. I would only open it once I was sitting comfortably on my sofa with a cup of tea at hand. Slowly I read it, starting with words that I have heard many times from so many people at various periods in my life, 'Charlotte, you have created chaos in my life.' Just like all the other times, I became sensitive and insecure but I continued reading. As I continued I felt a glow filling my whole body; even my useless limbs felt more alive. Stig wrote that he had told his wife about us. They had now initiated divorce proceedings. I could only imagine his intense blue-grey eyes filled with pain because he was splitting up his family. He eventually ended his letter by telling me to be patient. As a surprise, a few days later Stig called me. "Charlotte, I am sorry for this mess. We both need to be as patient as possible, it is very difficult for me, too. I need you to pull back a little." I listened without replying and he continued. "I am worried about my two sons. It is a tough time they are going through."

Finally, I reacted. "Sure, I will be patient and wait to hear from you." (Even though I only wanted to ask him, 'What about me?')

It was 20 August, four months after I woke up from my coma. A lot of things had happened in my new life. I was back at work, I had my own home but I still had not heard from Stig. During my lunch break that day, Stig suddenly called.

"Charlotte, how are you? I am able to come and visit you the first weekend in September." I felt a big smile grow on my face and a river of warm blood run through my body.

"Wonderful, Stig. I am okay. I am so looking forward to seeing you! But I have invited my class for a sleepover from Friday the second. So maybe it would be better if you arrived on Saturday?"

In that second I did consider cancelling their visit but I knew they would be so disappointed. So I did not suggest it; luckily, because Stig's reaction was a suprise.

"No problem. In that case I will arrive late on the first to help with the preparations."

I was so crazy about that man. On my return to the classroom after the break I told the children the news that my boyfriend would be with us for the sleepover. Just hearing myself call him boyfriend gave me again a warm feeling inside.

Stig arrived on the first in the late afternoon as promised. Again he had a large box in his arms. This time it was full of food. It turned out he knew what children liked and how to keep all twelve of them occupied. He had purchased cake mix, lemonade, crisps and plenty of paper towels for the inevitable mess. We spent a busy evening together making cakes and buns and all of the time talking and planning activities for the children.

Despite all of our preparations the sleepover became a bigger challenge than I had initially anticipated. By the time they had all arrived and we were sitting down drinking the lemonade and eating cake, I was exhausted. The children clearly sensed that I was already tired. So they tried to help with practical things such as laying the table and serving more helping of cake and lemonade, and even clearing up for me afterwards. We played bingo and checkers before sitting down to a meal of spaghetti and meatballs. Afterwards, we went out to the school playground for a final game of treasure hunt before bed. At about 10 pm and after the fourth or fifth time of telling them to shut up and go to sleep, I was almost crying with tiredness and ready for bed myself. Next morning after breakfast they were ready to go home, happy and content. I was just thankful that I had had Stig to help.

"Maybe it would be better if you took a short break to relax before throwing yourself back into the labour market again." They were the first words I heard from Stig after we had put the house back in order. I had just told him that I would take a short nap. Every muscle in my body and every one of my brain cells agreed with him. I was just too proud and stubborn to admit it. He was right. I was afraid to admit to myself that it was hard work. Because if I did, I would be admitting to myself that I was a failure; although it was only five months since my brain haemorrhage. I kept telling myself that I should be capable of working. I let myself fall into his arms and asked him: "Who am I, if I am not the teacher?"

He laughed at me and answered quickly, "You are still Charlotte. You just need some time out to decide exactly what it is that you want to do with the rest of your life."

29

Bonus children

I continued my work at the school until the autumn break in October 1989, six months after I had had my brain haemorrhage. It was becoming harder for me to get out of bed in the mornings because my body was sore and tired. Every day I returned home from work and needed to have a short sleep. It was a terrible time for me. Everything in my heart told me to continue and create a normal life for myself, but in my head I knew that my body still needed time to recover.

On the day that the school closed for the ten days' holiday I told the headmaster that I needed some sick leave. Later that day I travelled with my parents to visit my sister in France. It was the same day Stig and his two sons moved out of their home and into an apartment at the hospital complex in Viborg.

The trip to France did not start well. We had not even

crossed the border into Germany before Mum opened the picnic hamper and brought out lunch. She had, of course, made all of my favourites; hard-boiled eggs with mayonnaise, tomato and cucumber and fishcakes with pickles all neatly decorated with thin slices of lemons and cucumbers. Beautiful to look at but not very easy to eat with only one hand and sitting in a shaking bus at the same time. Before I had finished the first tomato sandwich I was covered in its juice. By the time I had the egg mayonnaise sandwich I was a mess. After lunch I needed to go to the toilet to clean up. The toilet was situated in the centre of the bus and we were at the front. As I stood up I looked quickly at my sticky T-shirt and greasy fingers. I promptly fell backwards onto the lap of the lady sitting next to me. I could not maintain my balance in the moving vehicle. I was flushing red with embarrassment and could feel the eyes of my fellow travellers watching me. I had no choice but continue to play my part in this comedy of errors, and made my way towards the toilet. Not content with just looking a mess, my body decided to go one step further with the entertainment. Just as I reached the narrow door my left arm suddenly went into cramp mode and slammed itself up under my chin.

Eventually, we arrived at my sister's house. I soon gave myself up to her sincere care and let myself be waited on hand and foot. I followed her around with her daily routine such as the school run and daily shopping. Each time we went by car I was so happy . She had a BMW cabriolet. When I sat in the passenger seat next to her and felt the breeze through my hair, no one could see my floppy arm or crooked walk. All they saw were two young women out for a drive seemingly without a care in the world.

Any doubts that I might have had about my relationship with Stig were pushed aside. When we were on our way home from France, I stopped off at Viborg to see him and his new home. He introduced me to his sons as his girlfriend. I felt happy in the knowledge that he wanted both his sons and me in his life. Stig had prepared a dinner for us and during the meal I managed to score a lot of cheap points by telling Stig that teenage boys needed to visit the hairdressers at least once a month. Also that their jeans had to be American 'Levis'. The boys were very nice and welcoming to me. I was nice to them, too, but I got very tired of their constant chatter. My only real experience of children was at school. There I could take frequent breaks from the noise. After several later visits to Stig I began to get used to having the boys around and found that I was enjoying their company more and more. I must admit when they were away visiting their mother and I had Stig to myself, it was much better. As time passed I spent more of my time with Stig. We decided that it would be better for me to give up my little house and move in with them. In December 1989 I left my house in Åbyro and moved to their apartment in Viborg. I now had the man of my dreams and two bonus teenage sons, but no job. It was during this period that, for the first time, I probably, started to listen to what my body was telling me. When my brain told me to rest, I did. So I slept up to fourteen hours a day. To this day, I have no idea how Stig managed to cope with me either in bed or lying over the sofa as he worked to create a stable home for his two sons. During these months I contributed nothing either physically or financially to our little family.

30

My new career

After about six months I felt that I had energy again and I could start to be an active member of our household.

I got in touch with my social worker in Viborg and made arrangements to meet in her office. As I arrived, she gave me a lookover before saying with a smile, "For a strong, young woman like you, it is time to get back to work." Her words were like honey to my ears and I could have cried with happiness on hearing them. She gave me the motivation and I was ready to co-operate with her in any way to make a rehabilitation plan for myself. We had a few meetings to develop the plan. I would retrain as a special needs teacher. At the same time she would try to find me work as an intern in various centres for adults. I would then spend a year at the university in København learning to be a special reading therapist. I loved the plan.

We moved from the apartment in the hospital to

another on the third floor in the city centre. Climbing the stairs became part of my daily exercise. The feeling of regaining more control over my body was so important for me. I would say in that period exercising became like a drug for me.

One evening we were collecting Stig's son from his karate lessons when I met his coach, Jens, a man who was to become a fascinating and significant part of my life. Jens was a former bodybuilder. His height of two metres and his muscular frame were at odds with his delicate way of walking. It seemed as if he was tiptoeing as he walked round the gym. As the owner of the fitness complex where some of the biggest bodybuilders in the town worked out, Jens was always in great demand. During his free time he ran the karate school where he taught both the physical form of the Japanese art and the philosophy behind it. As if this wasn't enough and this was more important to me, he and his staff specialised in training disabled people. For this reason he had created a small club for the disabled. I recall his first words to me that evening.

"I think that we have some exercises that may be of some interest to you."

My response was immediate. "That I doubt very much."

I looked around the room and saw men with muscles on muscles lifting weights. In the next room skinny girls in pink leotards were doing aerobics. Jens just looked at me, laughing.

"Come back tomorrow at 10 am. If you don't have

any gym clothes just stay for coffee. But leave your prejudices at home."

It was a challenge I had to take.

So at 10 am the next morning I returned with suitable clothing. A few hours later when I eventually left the centre, I was so tired, physically exhausted from the exercise and amazed by the positive impressions that I received from the disabled people in the group. After exercising I had a coffee with the group. The togetherness with them was very close and the conversation was free, open-minded and confident. Jens was right and I quickly became a member of the club and went to the centre almost every day. I had a great sense of satisfaction from my time at the gym and also the time I spent with the others in the group. I still did not identify myself with the group as 'disabled' but more with our common life situations as being a mixed bunch of characters in a streamlined community, which surely tells you more about me than the rest of them.

Jens' philosophy regarding our training was to make us focus on the physical skills we still had rather than the ones we did not. This was a new and constructive way of looking at myself and a way of thinking that I could directly translate to the courses and internships that I intended to join as part of my own rehabilitation plan. Slowly I managed to change my focus away from what did not work for me to what did and gave me energy. I returned to my social worker and told her that I was ready for work. I wanted a job where I could use my education as a teacher while making use of my personal experiences as a disabled young woman. She quickly found me my first internship at the rehabilitation unit's school for special needs. The very one that I visited while staying at the physiotherapy rehabilitation unit. I was to shadow the two teachers, Anita and Erna.

Instead of welcoming me, Anita just gave me a look and said, "Now we understand your interest in Stig when you were here as a patient."

Erna continued, "We know already that you know how to teach. Forget about being a shadow and get to work .With five students here today we need you!" I smiled at Anita, looked directly at Erna and said, "Just tell me what to do. I am ready!"

Luckily for me, Stig was no longer working at the rehabilitation unit but had changed to a consulting job out of the hospital.

The first day at work I arrived in the pouring rain. I found it very difficult to rediscover my enthusiasm for the place. Almost as soon as the large sliding doors closed Lasse saw me and called me over.

"Charlotte, please come over and help me convince my patient that it pays to fight and keep on working at his exercise."

I had to force myself to concentrate and walk as easily as possible towards the young man standing as stiff as a tree between the parallel bars. I smiled at him.

"Lasse is right. It pays off. Look at me. A year ago it was me standing where you are. Now I am back to work here."

As I turned around to walk away, I heard the young man behind me. "Wow"

Later in the classroom when I was sitting with my first student, I remembered the positive atmosphere in this nice room with the beautiful view over the lake even though it was raining. For the first time in a long while I felt like a normal person. I had something to offer other adults. Besides teaching the physically disabled, I started to teach mentally ill adults and others with acquired brain injuries.

I had to go to København for the training I needed to be a special reading therapist for adults with language problems. As most of the courses were on Fridays or at the weekend I could work for the Viborg social services during the week. I counselled over the phone young, disabled people. I was lucky that Stig was taking care of everything at home. I was either working, studying or sleeping. It was an incredibly exciting and educational time in my life both professionally and personally.

31

Bride to be

I had no doubt about my answer when Stig proposed to me. I was surprised that he would want to marry a young, disabled woman. I could not stop thinking how, in my situation, I deserved to be so lucky and happy. It was these thoughts that made me ask for the wedding to take place before the end of 1990. I was so afraid that he might change his mind if we waited any longer. Stig was so old-fashioned. On our next visit to my parents he asked my father for my hand in marriage. We were sitting in the garden behind their house drinking coffee when Stig suddenly said, "Børge, I would like to ask your permission to marry Charlotte." Slowly and with great deliberation my father took a sip from his cup and looked over at Stig. I tried to read the look on my father's face but he was a blank canvas to me. My mother's face on the other hand lit up like a Christmas tree. I struggled to try to come up with an idea of what my father was thinking right now. I knew that my father thought he and Stig were polar opposites. Stig was an intellectual from the capital and he himself a man from the country who left school after seven years and supported his family by manual labour. Anyhow, my father also knew that they had an invisible bond in a common love for me. Besides, they had both eaten boiled pigs' trotters in jelly when they were children!

My father drank again before he answered Stig.

"So, you want to marry my Charlotte. I suppose I can always dig up some potatoes and leeks that we can eat at the reception."

Stig looked a bit confused but managed to smile and whispered, "Thank you!"

He did not understand what I knew. It was my father's way of telling Stig that my father was going to pay for the wedding party. I explained this to Stig the next day.

"Do not worry, Stig. We do not need to eat potato and leeks at the wedding. It was just my father's way of telling you that he will pay for everything."

Stig laughed loudly and left the room. When he came back he showed me a copy of the letter he had sent to the American Embassy. He had made a request for us to be married in the town of Charlotte Amalia, the capital of one of the small American Virgin Islands. I looked at him and said, "How romantic but I do not think my father will pay for this." The financial arrangements after Stig's divorce changed these plans. Stig accepted my father's offer. We decided to hold the service in the little church just outside Løgstør and the priest who would perform the ceremony would be the same one who had baptised me twenty-six years earlier.

The day of the wedding, 29 December 1990, turned out to be the coldest day of winter that year. Much to the surprise of some of my friends I chose to wear a vintage wedding dress from Paris that would cover my peculiar way of walking. Just to make certain that their eyes were looking away from the ground I borrowed a big hat to complement the dress.

To buy the shoes that went with my outfit proved to be very difficult.

Because of my paralysed foot I could not wear any of the usual shoes found in bridal shops and after a month's searching I was getting desperate. No way was I going to wear training shoes for my wedding even though they were the most comfortable for me. Frustrated by the saleswomen in the wedding shops who never listened to me – they only offered me high-heeled and narrow, pointed-toe shoes – I gave up and went to Aalborg to a 'normal' shoe shop where I met the most sensitive woman. She must have had at least twenty-five years' experience in shoe selling.

"Please tell me your size and then walk up and down the floor a couple of times."

I did and said, "I am a size 38."

She smiled. "I think for you last year's model 'Ecco' summer shoe would be the best. It has a low heel and is wide fitting but it is still a very elegant shoe." She and her colleague disappeared into the back storeroom where after a little time she returned with a very battered shoebox. Fortunately the contents were intact and they turned out to be just perfect for me.

On my wedding day I was at the house of Lotte's parents where my sister and Lotte were helping to dress the bride. With my half-length red hair washed and styled and my make-up on, they helped me into the dress and shoes. Up until that moment I had studiously ignored the full-length mirror in the room. Now it was time to look into it. Unable to help myself I say out loud: "I look normal!" "Whatever normal is," answered Lotte from behind me.

My sister laughed loudly. "You do not know, Charlotte! During high school you tried so hard not to be normal. Now it turns out that all you want in life is to be normal."

Like most brides I was filled with feelings of excitement and joy as I held on tight to my father's arm as we walked down the aisle. Near the altar Stig turned to look at me and I saw nothing else, just the brightest grey-blue eyes smiling at me. As my father and Stig's best man changed places Stig leaned in and whispered to me. "Darling, you don't have to sing the hymns." I struggled not to laugh. I was not very good at singing. I couldn't sing in tune even if my life depended on it. In that second I knew he wanted me. All of me!

I was enjoying my new married life with Stig and his two sons. I was being challenged daily by them. I might not have had the stretch marks or nappies to wash. Instead I did witness their first pimples, the first time they came home drunk and the first heartbreak. Stig and I did consider having our own child. We agreed quickly that I was working overtime both physically and mentally with my life. So to have a child as well would be too much for us to cope with. I was very lucky with Stig's sons in that I could let them fulfil my need for children. I never had to act as a second mother to them. I had absolutely no idea how to be a mother. I imagined it must be something wonderful to experience the unconditional love and at the same time feel the huge sense of responsibility that goes with having a baby. As I experienced neither, I chose a more practical approach to our new little family. I told the boys to look at our new little family as one where we were four different people each with different needs and where we had to respect and take care of each other. At the same time I understood that me moving in with them had changed their lives in many ways. I was full of admiration and appreciation for the way they welcomed me into their lives. I was now a wife and a bonus mother.

32

Life companions

Five years after I met Stig and had my brain haemorrhage Stig transferred his work to the hospital in Sønderborg. It was wonderful to start over. Everything would have been all joy and happiness if it were not for the fact that Stig had a heart attack on the day we were to move into our new home. For a long period our roles were reversed. I was responsible for our family and home. It was a challenge for me. Luckily, I now had more physical and mental energy and could manage with the change of position, although I did ask Peter and Marie for some help with the practical side of setting up our new apartment. It gave me the time to return to Viborg to be at the hospital with Stig. It was during this period of his illness that I became much closer to his sons. No longer boys, they were now young men of eighteen and twenty and soon to leave home to make their own way in the world.

The heart attack was soon followed by a second. As if that wasn't enough, diabetes was diagnosed. After a heart bypass operation, Stig was finally released from hospital. Once he was fully recovered we decided that we should take a short holiday on one of the Greek islands. We eventually arrived at our destination. Once we had settled ourselves in our room we decided to ask the receptionist for directions to the best beach. It turned out that we had a walk of over two kilometres on a bumpy dust road under the warm Greek sun. Finally we arrived and were soaked with sweat and exhausted as we had been running a 'Dream Mile'. But when we looked around us we saw a beautiful bay with golden sand and clear blue sea. Just the sight gave us new energy. Probably because it was such a long way from any of the hotels and not many tourists would want to walk that far, there were no sunbeds and umbrellas for us to rent. We had to spread ourselves out on the sand in the shadow of some large rocks that formed the backdrop of our beach.

Lying there I decided to lean in and give Stig a kiss. It proved to be more difficult than romantic. Stig was on my left, which of course was my paralysed side. I'd have to get up and change sides if I wanted to kiss him. With some help from him I managed to manoeuvre myself to the other side. Finally, I was back on the warm sand close to my husband and able to raise myself to kiss him but all my moving around had killed my intention of being romantic. Now even more exhausted, we both drifted off into a light sleep.When I woke I looked over at Stig at the long scar running down his chest. I ran my index finger gently over it as he woke. The scar and loss of twenty kilos in weight was the visible evidence of his long illness and successful operation. I leaned over and gently kissed him again.

"Look at us. We have become a pair of cripples," he said with a smile on his lips. Slowly I lifted myself up and leant against the rock.

"We are not a pair of cripples," I responded indignantly. "We are a cool couple. We have to agree that disease will never define our lives or become our identities. It can only be our life companions. Agreed?"

It was on one of the last days of our holiday when we joined a day trip with a large group that I had my little incident, which gave me cause to think about my disability; not least because of Stig's reaction to it. We had taken a bus to a large and beautiful beach. There were many people standing close together in the shallow water. Maybe because I was hot in the sun and my feet were in the cold water but my left arm reacted with a sudden spasm and contracted up against my chin; much to the surprise and shock of the Dutchman standing next to me. My hand caught the hem of his baggy shorts and yanked them upwards. Such a sudden and violent action caused them to pull tightly into his testicles. He pulled quickly away from me and readjusted his shorts to get comfortable again. I was scarlet with embarrassment at what had just happened to him. I gave him a huge smile when I tied to explain.

"I am so sorry! It was not me but me paralysed arm!"

He glared at me and ran further into the water. I guessed it was to get away from the mad woman. I turned to Stig for some comfort. But heard him say loudly, "This arm is not only attached to you, Charlotte. It is you!"

In my heart I knew that he was right. Even so, sometimes I felt that it was not a part of my body. It was a lifeless excrescence that grew on me like a parasite.

33

More sickness

The young doctor seemed either extremely nervous or very insecure as she opened the consultation in a very awkward way. She started off by saying: "I am glad that you have brought your family with you today, Stig."

Stig, his oldest son and I all looked at her. "Because you are going to tell me that I have a malignant carcinoma of the oesophagus." Stig's interruption made her look up at us quickly. Whether she was scared or relieved by his interruption I did not know.

Her reply was a short and sharp, "Yes!"

Stig's son then asked, "What is that?"

Before the doctor could explain Stig turned to his son and answered. "It is a malignant cancer tumour at the bottom of my oesophagus. It was the reason why I could not swallow food on our trip." Stig and his son had recently returned from a cycling tour of the Camino area in Spain.

When I heard those words, it made my blood run cold and my head stopped taking in any more information. I believed that we said goodbye shortly after and returned to the car in a shocked silence. Stig's son took his place behind the wheel of the car, me in the passenger seat and Stig in the back seat. I was the first to break the silence by asking, "Can you please drive me to work?"

His son looked over to me in silence and shook his head. From the back seat of the car Stig answered. "Of course we can."

In my head I mumbled a quick 'Thank you' and hoped that Stig understood the reason I was running away at this moment. I was thirty-eight years old. Thirteen years had passed since my brain haemorrhage and there was no more space in my head or life for any more illness. I needed to be somewhere that I could be in control. I knew it could only be at the school. Here I could hide behind teaching plans and hiring more temporary staff. Stig had to go to the university hospital in Odense for the operation. I was, of course, with him all of the time. I did not once think about the school or any of the problems there. It was not until three weeks later when we returned home from Odense, and I returned to work, that I finally started to feel a sense of normality again.

This was probably the reason that I did not listen to Stig when he, one evening, said to me, "Charlotte, I think you are suffering from stress."

I turned and looked him directly in his eyes. "Me! No way!"

He smiled. "I see you when you wake up in the middle of the night to take notes."

I looked down. "Okay, but I do not get out of bed."

"No, because you now have a notepad and a pencil on your bedside table. Besides, I can see that you have started to get several abdominal pains." A couple of weeks later I had to sign off sick from work with stomach ulcers. It was at the same time Stig retired for health reasons. The cancer had gone but the operation had left him without his oesophagus and only half a stomach. The doctor who released him said, "Stig, you are not going to die from cancer but probably slowly from hunger. Go home. Apply for your pension and enjoy your life with Charlotte."

Although we were having a wonderful time together at home, I was getting impatient to return to school again. As soon as I was back working, I felt happy. With my salary I was now able to contribute to household expenses. It made me feel both equal and independent. My working time was now the reverse to when I was in Åbybro and Aalborg before I had my my brain haemorrhage. My days were much longer and the nights shorter, which meant that I had less time to spend with Stig. He was the one that did everything in the house and made me dinner. Almost every night after dinner we sat on the sofa to watch the television and I inevitably fell asleep.

I remembered one particular Friday. We were at a

friend's house for dinner. After a delicious meal we moved onto the sofa for a last bottle of wine before going home. It was not long into the conversation before I could feel my eyelids beginning to drop. I struggled to keep my eyes open and follow the conversation. I kicked off my shoes and pulled my feet up under me. I ate chocolate just to try to keep myself awake. A few moments later I gave up. I allowed myself the luxury of a short break and closed my eyes for a second. The voices of Stig and our friends faded in my head before they disappeared completely. I was asleep. The next thing I knew Stig was slapping me hard on the leg and I woke up. Flustered, I started to apologise.

"Sorry, it has been a very busy week!"

My friend answered without looking at me. "Charlotte, I think most of your weeks are busy. I look forward to the day when you understand that work is not the only way to identify yourself!"

34

Work, work, work

In my mind I did not understand what our friend meant about work and identity. I continued to work at the same speed. A few weeks later I began my training to be a special reading therapist in København, which I did on top of my teaching. It meant I was now working at the weekends as well. I was fully occupied and it seemed that Stig was the only one to understand me. At least he did not complain. Once Stig had recovered from his cancer operation and was okay, I felt my ambitions starting to resurface. I finally graduated as a reading therapist. I managed to find full-time work at an evening school but every day I scanned the employment advertisements.

One day I saw a position advertised for a Danish teacher at a nearby boarding school. Immediately I telephoned the school to talk about the position. I will never forget the last part of our conversation.

"I have a paralysed arm."

His reaction shocked me. "I do not think that you should be applying for this position."

This stupid, arrogant, ignorant man had in those few words made me feel like a second-rate teacher. In spite of my qualification he had discarded me just because I had a physical disability. I knew I was a good teacher. Certainly, I still wanted to teach. I also knew that teaching adults did not tax me physically and it did not challenge me. I really missed working with children. I missed their spontaneity and their openness to new things.

A friend showed me an ad for a local school, Lysabild School. They were looking for someone to work as a teacher in a special class. It was a contradiction but I rejected the idea because of the risk of being confronted by their honesty. After second thoughts, I felt that I was being stupid. How could I miss their spontaneity and openness and be afraid of their honesty? I had gained both mental and physical strength together with a stronger voice since my early days in Åbybro. It was a new challenge that I had to set myself. The work was covering maternity leave and so if it did not suit the school or the school did not suit me nothing would be lost. This time I did not draw attention to my arm when I arrived at the school for my interview with the headmaster, and neither did he. We talked for over an hour about the position and teaching in general. Eventually, I thought we needed to talk about me being paralysed. I raised the subject.

"Maybe you have not noticed it but the left side of my body is partially paralysed."

He looked up. "I noticed it as soon as you arrived but I wanted to talk to the teacher and not be confined to the shell she inhabits. Furthermore, from our talk now and your attitude, I am thinking that you may prefer to have the job as head teacher. If that's the case, you will be spending most of your time sitting behind a desk and your paralysed arm will not be a problem."

I laughed loudly. How could this man read my ambitions so clearly?

Lysabild School turned out to be a fantastic place to be. It had a very relaxed and open-minded atmosphere. From the very first day I felt at home. I started as a temporary teacher working alongside another teacher in a newly established special class for children diagnosed as having general learning difficulties, socio-emotional problems and ADHD; in my opinion, a bit of a catch-all. The teacher I was covering for never did return to work though, and so I applied for the position as permanent teacher. Every day I experienced incredible satisfaction. It turned out that being physically disabled meant I could use it to my advantage with most of the pupils. Often I had to ask them for practical help which gave them a small but significant boost to their own self-esteem.

One morning I received a phone call from one of the parents telling me that their son had been awake most of the night feeling sick. Nevertheless, he had said to her, "I have to go to school, because Charlotte needs my help."

I explained to the mother, "As you probably know, I

have some physical difficulties. So I ask the children to help me with some of the smaller tasks. I want to try and give them a sense of responsibility and of being needed despite having their own problems. Of course, I will call you if he is taken ill during the day."

From the start the second teacher and I shared the position of form teacher but it soon became clear to me it was not enough. I needed more of a challenge and more responsibility for our group. I asked my colleague about the possibility of being the only one in charge. Fortunately she agreed to let me take over the day-to-day running of the class. She would help with the putting forward of new ideas and plans. It was from that small step everything started to gather momentum. Within a couple of years we had expanded into a full-support department with a class for each educational diagnosis and had after-school facilities. We were still within the Lysabild School but now employed another thirteen people.

After discussing it with my colleagues, I addressed myself to the chief executive of the social services. I suggested to him that I be appointed director of the full-support department. This was something that he did not immediately agree with. So I asked him, "Is it because of my disability?" I looked him directly in his eyes. He looked back with a big smile on his face. "Your only disability in my eyes is your wilful nature." He quickly continued, "No, money is the problem. I will need to wait until the council can work out a new budget."

True to his word, by the time we had the new school

year planned, it was sorted out. I had a new title and new responsibilities.

Now I was working most days from early morning until late afternoon. I did not teach very much. I had to take care of all the administration and meetings with co-operates such as social workers, psycholgists and parents. Besides that, I became a governor of Lysabild School. I loved my work. It seemed at last that I had attained my never-articulated goals. I had proved to myself and people around me that not only could I return to teaching, I could become the head of a new full-support department. I was satisfied but also extremely tired.

When I was asked to extend my work with family counselling to include the parents of pupils from our department, I was proud and happy to take on a new challenge, even though it meant a new education as a family counsellor in the Netherlands. Fortunately for me I had my loving husband behind me. He gave me his support and help. He understood or at least accepted my constant need to prove to myself and others that I was capable of fulfilling any task that I set my mind to.

Part of my job as a family counsellor was counselling in the field. When a socially vulnerable family needed help, I went to their home to visit them three or four times for at least two hours at a time for them to gain trust in me and feel comfortable with me. Then I went once to make a video of their daily life situation. It could be them having dinner together on a school night or something similar. I did a thirty-minute video, analysed it and returned to show the parents everything they did right with their children. Often then they pointed out themselves what they did wrong.

On my third visit to a family with two children, a girl aged six and a son aged ten, the father tried to explain something to me about his own childhood. While doing it, his son made fun of him because he pronounced a word wrong. The father got up from his chair, grabbed a big wooden spoon from a casserole on the stove and tried to hit his son in the face. He did not but the warm brown sauce dripped on his son's hair. Next to me, his wife screamed loudly. I tried to stay calm and I said to myself: *What can I do? I cannot hit him or even run away because of my paralysed leg.*

The wife screamed to her husband. "Stop it, you stupid man!"

He turned around towards her. "Shut up. I will not listen to him or you insulting me!"

Then I knew I had to do something and I rose from the chair and found the courage to look the father in the eyes and said, "Maybe you will listen to me? If you hit your son, I will report it to the social services and to the police. According to Danish law you are not allowed to hit your children."

I could fell my legs shaking and my palms getting wet with sweat. I took a short pause. "Please sit down and let us talk."

He sat down, looked at me and surprisingly answered, "You, I will listen to you, because I think you, as a disabled person, know about being insulted."

I did not comment on his remark but sent a thought

to my friend from the Friday-night dinner. How could this job not be at least part of my identity?

Often I did not go home between my schoolwork and my visits to the families. So I spent a lot of time in my office at the school. One day, at a meeting in our unit, a colleague said to me, "Charlotte, it is nice that I always feel supported and understood if I call in sick. But it is a bit strange that you, as our leader, never calls in sick. You are always present. It kind of gives me a signal that I am weak because I call in sick." I understood what she meant.

I could only reply by telling her, "I am always here because I need to prove to myself that I can do my job. Besides, I am not very good at delegating responsibility."

I knew she had a point. I decided to talk to both Stig and my supervisor. During our talks I discover that my need to take control and to improve the department had been part of my need to prove to myself that I was capable. Now I had done it. I was ready to reconsider my situation. Shortly after, I told my collegues, "I am ready to relinquish my role as head of the department. I am going to work only as a family counsellor." It was not too long before I felt how good it was for my tired body. For a while my stomach pains disappeared. I also had time to resume my daily exercise routine. That was good for me physically. Unfortunately, my emotional side was telling me I had given in. Illness had won.

35

Tuscany

The light was overwhelming and was literally burning my eyes as I woke up. Sunlight was streaming through the open shutters of the windows of our hotel room. I pulled myself up into a sitting position from the big bed, resting my back against the cool stone wall that formed the headboard. Stig had opened the shutters when he returned from taking a shower. I turned my gaze from him and looked out of the window onto the beautiful Tuscany countryside where the trees and shrubs were either just coming into bud or were in full bloom. I smiled and whispered, "Every morning should start like this. It is pure vitamins for the soul."

Stig smiled back at me. "How about if we leave our predictable life in rainy Denmark and move to Tuscany?"

He had said something similar a few years earlier, when we were touring Tuscany on holiday with a couple of friends and were spending a few days in the historic centre of Lucca. It had been at lunchtime and we were sitting with a glass of beer in one of the many squares. I remembered Stig saying: "If it is going to be, it is going to be in Lucca!" At that time I did not think too much about it. I was too busy working to prove myself; to prove I was good enough. I never understood a seed had been planted. It had just taken some time to germinate.

It was now mid June, 2006, seventeen years after my brain haemorrhage. We were back in Lucca to celebrate Stig's sixtieth birthday. We and eighteen of our closest family and friends were all staying together in a small hotel just outside the ancient town. This time I was more than ready to go with his idea. I ran my hand over his knee to get his attention. When he looked me in the eyes I answered without hesitation. "Okay! Let's do it!" He smiled at me, understanding exactly what I meant with my cryptic remark and gave me a quick kiss. Next morning we sat propped up in bed with cups of coffee in hand and gave each other the ultimate challenge. We would make the move to Italy and live our lives without being defined by our work or health problems.

"I am no longer the teacher with a paralysed side. I am Charlotte, your wife," I said to Stig.

He replied quickly, "I am no longer the neuropsychologist. I am Stig, your husband."

Later that evening at the restaurant where we were hosting Stig's birthday dinner, Stig stood to make a short speech: "Thank you everyone for coming here to help me celebrate my sixtieth birthday. In future you will have to come to Lucca to see Charlotte and me. We have decided to move here and will be doing it within a year."

In February 2007, as Denmark was hit with a huge snowstorm, we arrived safely inside the protective walls of what was to be our new home city, Lucca. Squashed in our overloaded car between suitcases and boxes sat Charlie, our beloved dog. We were all ready to begin a new adventure. The reactions of various friends and relatives regarding our decision to move lock, stock and barrel to Italy were varied to say the least. Stig's two sons were looking forward to making the journey south to stay with us for free Italian holidays, although they were worried that we might be running away from prospective duties as grandparents. They had both married. Rasmus, the youngest, lived with his wife in Viborg; Mads, the eldest, with his wife and family in Sønderborg. Friends had mixed views. One even said: "Cool that you two are actually leaving Denmark." It made us both think about why it was more cool that we did it. Without doubt it was going to be a big challenge for us to exchange our very comfortable life in a well-functioning country to an unpredictable one in chaotic Italy. Our Italian language skills were negligible. If I was being honest, non-existent would be a better way of putting it. Some of the problems raised by moving to another country are practical ones. Where are we going to live? Can we keep our Danish car? How do we find a doctor? It turned out that these were easy to sort out. The difficult one was how could we be just

Charlotte and Stig twenty-four hours a day without work to separate us?

We began our new life in Tuscany the way most people dream of spending a summer holiday. We rented a rustic stone house on a hillside overlooking a beautiful river. The house was huge, built on three levels and had a large roof terrace. The ground floor was one large room with a huge open fireplace and a narrow iron staircase leading up to the first floor. This became for us the main living space because it had direct access to the garden through the kitchen and dining room and a sitting room with windows overlooking the countryside. Our bedroom and bathroom were also on this floor. Up another set of stairs was the top floor, which had two further bedrooms and a bathroom. This floor was only used when we had guests staying. For the first eight months it was used almost continually. The gardens had a large olive grove and Stig loved playing the farmer, working daily cutting wood for the fire, taking care of the lemon trees and going for long walks with Charlie over terrain which was impossible for me to walk. I spent most of the first six months just sitting in the garden staring at the river. Now that there was nothing for me to do I could feel how tired my body was. My new Italian doctor tried to convince me to apply for a Danish pension but I refused. "Charlotte, with your body you will never be able to work as a teacher again," she kept on saying as if I was deaf. Her words hurt me. The fact that I did not have the language skills to explain to her that I could not bear the thought of never having the opportunity to return to work in Denmark made me frustrated. The doctor performed a number of various tests to show me just how damaged my back, hips and right shoulder were. With the medical evidence and pressure from Stig, I eventually applied for and received my Danish disability pension. It was a relief to know that I was economically secure for the rest of my life. Unfortunately, I could not help feeling that I had failed. In my heart I knew that I had made the right decision but my head had problems accepting it. Now I had to start something new. I decided to learn Italian. We stayed in the stone house for more than a year before we gave in to reality. It was a beautiful house but for us not very practical. We moved inside the walls and rented a modern apartment in an old palazzo. Luckily for us it was very unusual as it had a small, enclosed garden. It was possible for Stig to have his lemon trees and other shrubs to tend. He grew herbs in pots which he dried and used in his cooking. As well as the garden he enjoyed his other passion, road cycling. Stig recovered as much as possible from the cancer operation where they had to remove half his stomach. Luckily his body took great pleasure in the warm climate and the 'Mediterranean diet'. I had also found that the warm climate was a great help for my damaged arm and leg as the muscles were more relaxed. In the summer we made the most of a friend's swimming pool for exercise and in the colder and wetter days of winter I used my stationary exercise bike and walked the medieval wall that surrounded Lucca. Plenty of physical exercise gave me the satisfaction of having more control over my body. I found that the more exercise I did, the less reliant I was on painkillers. I had decided it was not a road for me to go down. Although it sounded like a contradiction in terms, living inside the enclosed walls I felt free and independent. During our daily life here we had got to know many other foreigners who, like us, had uprooted to live the Italian life. Italy is a country where it was a way of living just to be present. The Italians call it: '*Il dolce fare niente*'– 'The sweetness of doing nothing.'

36

The Meltdown

I had just turned forty-five. Twenty years had passed since my brain haemorrhage. Peter and Marie were visiting us in Lucca. The day before they were due to leave for the drive back home Peter got a sharp pain in his back. Stig drove him to the emergency room at the local hospital where the doctor on duty gave him a painkilling injection and a pack of five for Marie to give him so that he could manage the long drive through Europe. On their return from the hospital they found Marie and me sitting out in our courtyard garden drinking coffee. They joined us but I could see my brother was in great pain. Maybe because of the pain he seemed a bit irritated. The garden was lovely and warm, heated by the spring sunshine, and full of flowers; big, waxy pink camellias, the thousands of small purple bougainvillea petals and the heady perfume of the wisteria. It was the perfect setting for conversation and just being together. I don't recall exactly what was said by whom, only that the subject was of being a parent. Maybe the fact that I had never had children of my own was the catalyst for what happened next? I don't know. Or if it was because I could not cope with my brother's sudden need for care and the fact that I was not able to be there for him, as he had been for me all those years? I still don't know. I remember he said something about me not knowing what it was to be a parent. Even though I agreed with him, his words hit me like a bullet and cut a big hole inside my body. I suddenly felt a deep loss for never having had a child of my own.

I felt the suppressed lump of anger and frustration coming to life again inside my crooked body. Quickly it filled up the hole inside me; this lump that had been created in me back in the classroom in Åbybro when I realised I was not the same person after my brain haemorrhage. For the last twenty years the lump had festered inside me. Now I felt that it had become too big for my weak body to contain and was ready to explode into the world. I had no idea what word or sentence lit the fuse but suddenly it exploded. First came the wave of acidic juices of anger because I had not been able to do everything I wanted to in life. I started to scream at Peter, Marie and Stig. I accused them of the most unimaginable things possible.

Hurriedly Stig stood up and put his arms round me. Instead of feeling comforted, I felt a thousand needles pierce my body, and his fingers burnt into my flesh. I lashed out with my right hand and my left arm cramped up under my cheek. I was so angry that my body was shaking. Then a wave of frustration hit me because of my physical limitations and pain. It all ended in a massive crying session which knocked out every other emotion. The three of them were now standing looking at me. I was unable to look them in the eyes because I knew that I would see sympathy and understanding. Turning towards Peter, Marie said: "Maybe we should leave and start the drive home today."

It was not for me to decide but I felt that by leaving she was letting me down. My reaction to her words came as gun fire. "If you want to go, you'd better go now. If you do, you shall never come back, ever!" I screamed at them. In spite of Marie's frightened look I continued, "You do not leave when life hurts. You get through it together!"

My screaming was subdued by heaving sobs of agony. Of course, I had been angry before that fateful evening in 1989. Since then I had more than once been surprised at just how angry I could be. I had even experienced anger as an inexhaustible supply of positive energy that had enabled me to function physically.

This was the first time since I was in the hospital that I felt completely helpless. It was a total meltdown for me physically and mentally. Afterwards, I was very tired and extremely embarrassed, but no longer angry. I just felt empty of any emotions. I needed sleep. In that second I discovered that I had been confronted with a new challenge in my life. I had to learn how to feel, accept and live with vulnerability. Since waking up from my coma on 20 April 1989 it was something I had not allowed myself to feel. That afternoon in our garden I had to thank God that my meltdown happened when I was together with people who I knew loved me and would not judge me. They would always be there for me.

Since that day I have been angry or frustrated a few times mostly about practical challenges but I have not had any more meltdowns.

37

Think again

One might think that after more than twenty years with illness as a life companion I would have learned to be tolerant of my body's weaknesses. Think again! It had only made me extremely bad at coping. The undergoing of endless tests for Stig in hospital resulted in a new regime of drugs and diet changes which just wore me out, as did sickness of family and friends. Recently, a dear friend told me that she would never turn to me for compassion. It hurt to hear but I did not make any protest as I knew she was right. I have to admit that I have despised people who have had the courage to show just how vulnerable they are. I know that this is not very sympathetic but I have to be honest with you readers, then with myself.

38

Goal met

It was a long way back through the safe and narrow tunnel of sleep. We were in our apartment in Lucca, 2014. It was twenty-five years after my brain haemorrhage. I kept trying to focus on the intense grey-blue eyes staring back into mine. A passionate kiss that brought me back to the first time Stig came to visit me in my little house in Åbybro. I opened my eyes, looked at Stig and remembered the last words of his beautiful speech made a few days earlier in the scout hut in Denmark:

"The man who can drive himself further once the effort gets painful is the man who will win. Such a man are you, Charlotte." I looked him in the eyes and smiled. In that precise moment I knew it had been so many years since thinking: *what if I had not been taken ill that evening*?

Looking around I could see all of my memories, the

ones that I kept safely stored in my iron box. They were spread all over our bed and were the evidence of me running my 'Dream Mile'. This run that has made me the woman I am today; happy, tired, sometimes vulnerable, but still Charlotte. My 'Dream Mile' in many ways had enriched my life. Anger had slowly evaporated and my energy was now coming from the joy I had in choosing to hold on to life and myself. Not only did I run my 'Dream Mile', it took me all the way to Tuscany. I had met my goal. Of course, I had felt pain but I had never let pain control me or my life. I got up from the bed and collected all of the letters and photographs. I put them carefully back into the box, locked it with the padlock and carried it back to the shelf in our storeroom. I called out to Stig, "I am hungry and more than ready for a glass or two of bubbles."

As he was already waiting, he answered immediately. "Okay, let's go then!"

We walked round to the corner of Piazza Cittadella where sits the statue of Giaccomo Puccini, one of the famous sons of Lucca. We found our usual table outside Osteria Tosca. During the last six years this restaurant had become one of our favourite places to eat. Flavia, the owner, had also become a good friend. As usual we shared a dish of *spaghetti vongole* first. Then Stig took an almost rare *bistecca* and I ordered the fish and as often before, the chef, Michele, had removed all of the bones before serving me. It was a warm spring night and all of the tables were full and so we were all sitting Italian-style close together. I noticed the woman sitting next to me because of the fantastic silk dress in a bold design of purple, grey and yellow.

"Charlotte, you are staring," Stig hissed at me and for once he was right. I could not help it. Not only the beautiful dress caused me to stare at her. It was also the way she moved. The waiter served her a plate of *bruschetta* and placed it gently in the centre of the table. She raised her hand but left it hanging in mid-air until her male companion said to her in English, "To the left-hand side of your wine glass." I looked up at him – strangely, I had not noticed him sitting opposite her. She gently moved her hand to touch the wine glass with the back of it before she lowered her hand until her thumb touched the wet tomatoes. Then she opened her hand fully and picked up one of the pieces of bread. It was swamped with chopped fresh tomatoes, basil and finely chopped garlic. I was mesmerised as I watched her slowly lift it and place it on the plate in front of her. Even though I knew that I shouldn't I had to ask her.

"Are you blind?"

Immediately she turned her head towards me and answered me in her clear English voice, "Yes, I am."

I looked her in the eyes. "But how did you buy such a beautiful dress?" I said without thinking.

"My husband, he chose it for me!"

I sensed her reply had a hard edge to it, which was what I probably deserved for being so forward. I looked over at Stig as it suddenly dawned on me that I had done exactly what for the last twenty-five years I had tried to avoid myself. I had only seen her as a disabled woman and not as the person she was.

39

I got mail

The year is 2016, twenty-seven years since my brain haemorrhage. I am in my fifties, having passed the silver wedding with both Stig and my paralysed arm, when I finally found the courage to tell my story and try to find Jesper.

Hi Jesper

I am not sure if you remember me but twenty-seven years ago we had dinner in a small Greek restaurant when I was suddenly taken very ill. You quickly called for an ambulance. Because of your rapid reaction you helped to save my life and for that I would like to give you my heartfelt thanks. If you do remember, and one day have the time, could you please tell me your version of the episode that evening in 1989.

Ever-thankful Charlotte

A few hours later I received the following reply from him.

Hi Charlotte

What a totally unexpected but absolute pleasant surprise to find your message in my mailbox. No, to be honest almost unreal.

Do I remember you? How could I ever forget you? Over the last twenty-seven years I have often thought about you and what happened to you.

My memory is a bit blurred so all I can say about that evening is you suddenly felt very bad so I called for an ambulance. Nothing very heroic.

Jesper

It is amazing for me to read the e-mail from Jesper even though I have not thought about him very often since my stay in hospital but ever since 12 April 1989, he has just been a secret hero in my memory.

In January 2016 I received a letter from one of my Danish readers asking me: 'What happened to the young man you were having dinner with the evening you were taken ill?' Her question filled me with the desire to find him and thank him for his part in saving my life. I wrote a message on my Facebook page asking for anyone with any information about a man called Jesper who would be about fifty to fifty-five years of age and who had studied international economics in Aalborg in 1989. I said I would like to thank him for helping to save my life. Two days later I received a message from a former colleague in Sønderborg. She told me that she knew him and passed on his e-mail address so that I could write to him myself which I did. During the next couple of months we wrote each other several e-mails talking about our lives now and for the past twenty-seven years. The Danish version of my story was published and Jesper got a copy then I did not hear from him for some months. Then I received this e-mail.

Dear Charlotte

I want to thank you for taking the effort to find me. I have spent the last months trying to recall what happened in the Greek restaurant back in 1989. It has been quite a journey for me to get a hold on that dramatic experience. I will try to give you my version.

I remember we met, sat down and looked at the menu. You went to the bathroom and when you returned I noticed that you staggered a little bit. You sat down on the bench again and asked

197

me. "Do I look strange to you?" Quickly I denied it. After all, we were on our first date.

Then I realised that your face had changed. It had become loose on the left side. Your mouth and eye were hanging a bit so I knew something was wrong. I got up, went over to your side of the table and tried to make you lie down on the bench. You put up some resistance but I managed to persuade you.

"Please, put your legs up on the bench," I said. You lifted your right leg. "Fine, now the other leg."

You looked at me and I could see you did not understand which leg I was talking about. You thought you had taken up both your legs. By that time I knew something was seriously wrong and I left you to call for an ambulance.

Back in a second I saw that both your left leg and arm were hanging down from the bench. I took your left arm and placed your hand on your stomach but it would not stay. Immediately it fell down again.

Yes, I got the chance to be in the front of an ambulance. I do not know how I feel about that experience.

I was not allowed to stay at the hospital so I gave them my phone number and left.

High on adrenalin I went to see a friend as I needed to share what had happened. We had some beers which helped me to relax.

Back in my apartment there were several messages on my answering machine, all from your parents. They wanted me to come back to the hospital. So in the middle of the night and a bit drunk, I met your parents. What an impression they must have had of me.

Jesper

Reading his mail fills me with gratitude. It also gives me a feeling of being very close to this man I hardly know and have not seen for twenty-seven years but who, in this moment, I recall clearly. I remember our first meeting. I see him sitting on the sofa in Debora's apartment dressed in jeans and blue polo shirt with his brown hair, round, rosy cheeks and blue eyes. I can almost smell him. I know now that in my subconscious mind I wanted to find him to have him as my witness. I wanted him to fill in the gaps in my memory. This is the perfect closure for me.

My name is Charlotte and this is my story. Life can be difficult and fragile but we need to hold on to it gently because we never know just how fragile until it is too late.

Thank you

To write this book has been like doing another 'Dream Mile' and I couldn't have done it without help and support.

First of all, my English friend Stephen Hickman who patiently transformed my simple school English to a legible English so my Australian friend Jane Cutter could help me with the structure of my story and the final read done by Louise Fiona Aglioni. Then all those friends reading bits and parts through the process.

Also, a big thank you for all the kindly help from the staff at The Book Guild.

Finally, a huge thank you to the love of my life, my husband, Stig. He is my daily inspiration.